WELCOME

We often shy away from prioritising our health and wellbeing – whether that's because we're too embarrassed to talk about certain things or we're too busy juggling work, childcare, relationships, domestic chores and an attempt to have a social life. Often, hobbies and health are put on the back burner. Many of us also come from a long line of parents or caregivers who didn't feel comfortable talking about bodies or sex, let alone mental health. That's why we've decided to go back to basics and start at the very beginning! Once you've explored the female anatomy and found out exactly what happened to your body during puberty, we're going to take you on a journey that delves into a whole range of women's health issues. Understand the role of essential hormones; discover the importance of fitness and nutrition; and become more in tune with your mental health. We explain everything you need to know about menstrual cycles, ovulation and pregnancy, and look in-depth at sexual health and intimacy. We examine common health conditions, from diabetes and arthritis to endometriosis and fibroids, as well as gynaecological cancers and breast health. Discover how to look after your bowel and bladder, and what to expect in later life, including menopause and taking care of your bones, joints and heart. We also consider common procedures, essential screenings and inclusive healthcare.
Being a woman isn't always easy, and some things are out of our control, but knowledge is power, so turn the page and get to know yourself better today!

Disclaimer
This publication is for information only and is not intended to substitute professional medical advice and should not be relied on as health or personal advice. Never disregard professional advice or delay seeking it. Always consult your doctor or pharmacist for guidance and before using any natural, over-the-counter or prescription remedies, and read any instructions carefully. In an emergency, call the emergency services and seek professional help immediately. Readers rely on any information at their sole risk, and *The Healthy Woman's Handbook*, and its publisher, Future Publishing Ltd, limit their liability to the fullest extent permitted by law.

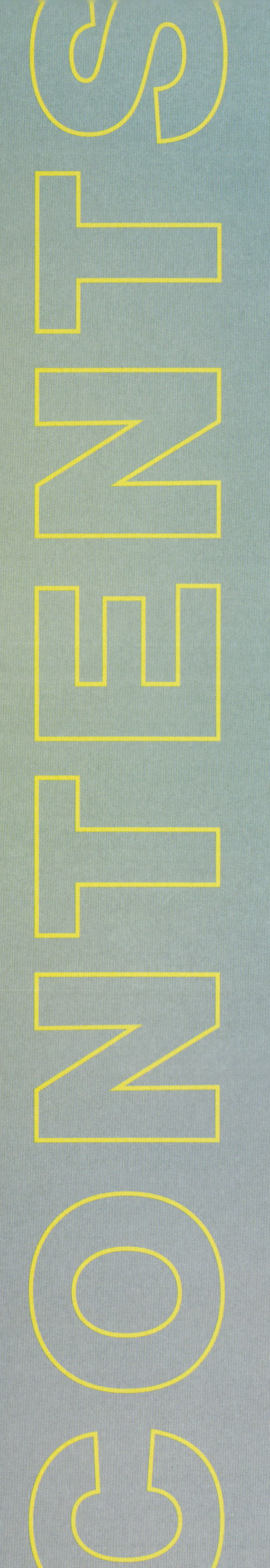

CONTENTS

6
Welcome To Your Healthy Woman's Handbook

8
The Female Anatomy

10
What Happens During Puberty?

16
A Guide To Essential Hormones

22
What Is Good Health?

28
Health Conditions

34
Fitness & Exercise

40
Diet & Nutrition

46
Mental Health In Women

50
Your Menstrual Cycle Explained

54
A Guide To Periods

58
What Impacts Ovulation

60
Contraception Options

62
Understanding Conception

66
A Guide To Pregnancy

72
Labour & Birth

76
Postpartum Health

80
Your Sexual Health

84
Intimacy, Libido & Emotions

88
Female Health Concerns

94
Gynaecological Cancers

100
Bladder, Urinary & Bowel Health

104
Breast Health

110
Common Procedures

114
Health Screenings

116
Inclusive Healthcare

118
Facing Menopause

124
Heart Health Post-Menopause

126
Bone & Joint Health

128
Understanding Dementia

WELCOME TO YOUR HEALTHY WOMAN'S HANDBOOK

Within these pages you will hopefully find all you need to know about your health and wellbeing

As a woman, our bodies change so much – from childhood and adolescence through to adulthood, and then into menopause and later life. Our health is determined by a complex balance of systems within our bodies, as well as the external influences that we're subjected to every day. Everything we experience, eat, drink, do and feel impacts on our health and wellbeing.

This title is designed to guide you through everything you need to know about your health. We go back to basics and explore the female anatomy, because the first step in being health-aware is knowing your own body inside and out. We're sure you've covered this all in your school biology lessons, but a refresher never hurts (especially if it's been a while!). And it helps to understand where everything is and what it does when it comes to learning more about health concerns and conditions.

For young girls, the first big change of life comes in at puberty, when hormone levels surge and bring out both physical and mental developments. You probably remember your own adolescent days and how hard it felt at times to come to terms with everything that was happening. Maybe you're now at the point when you have your own children or family members approaching the same stage of life. We explain what happens during this time and how it can influence your health as an adult.

Hormones are such a key part of the female experience. They have so much power over how we are physically and emotionally. We'll introduce you to the main hormones and you'll see how they play a part throughout your whole life, from puberty to reproduction to menopause. You will learn all about your menstrual cycle, periods and ovulation, to better understand how these systems all work. We have sections on conception, pregnancy and childbirth, as well as sexual function.

This book also looks at general health conditions and female-specific health conditions that you should be aware of, from simple infections through to more complex illnesses. We'll explain the warning signs, but we hope that you'll gain a new awareness of your body so that you can detect when something isn't right.

As with any guide, there will be sections of this book that are not relevant to you or don't quite match your situation. We've tried to be as inclusive as possible, but we can't cover every aspect of women's health. You can dip in to the sections that you need, when you need them. This guide is designed for women who want to learn more about their health and wellbeing, as well as for parents or caregivers to help explain or understand women's health in more detail. It can act as a jumping-off point to do more research in a specific area once you've mastered the basics.

We hope you find the advice and information in this book useful. ∎

> "THE FIRST STEP IN BEING HEALTH-AWARE IS KNOWING YOUR OWN BODY INSIDE AND OUT"

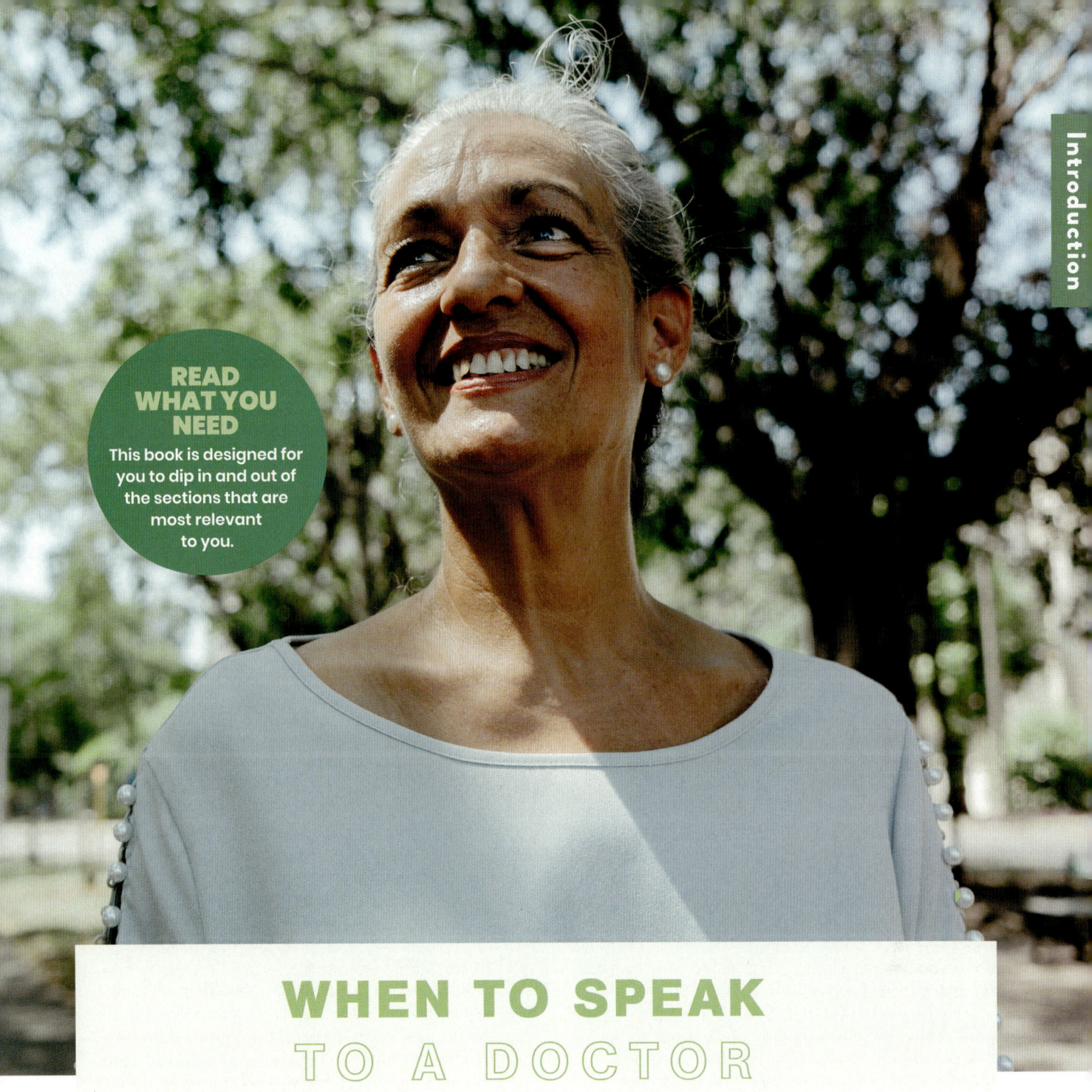

READ WHAT YOU NEED
This book is designed for you to dip in and out of the sections that are most relevant to you.

WHEN TO SPEAK
TO A DOCTOR

If you're worried about something to do with your health, seek medical advice

This book provides an overview of women's health, but it's not exhaustive. It shouldn't be used as medical advice. We present the information here to help you understand more about your body, how to look after it and some of the potential conditions or illnesses you may face along the way. We hope this guide proves useful in helping you to learn more about your health, but you should always trust your instinct. If something doesn't feel right, then always get a professional medical opinion. One of the benefits of getting to know your body and your health more deeply is that you're more in tune with how you feel. It means you may pick up on warning signs more quickly, which enables you to treat any problems as soon as possible. You should always see a doctor if you have unexplained weight loss, increased fatigue, chest pain, a cough that won't go away, persistent headaches, a lump or changes to your bowel habits. It's better to seek advice when it's not serious, than leave it and risk it being something worse.

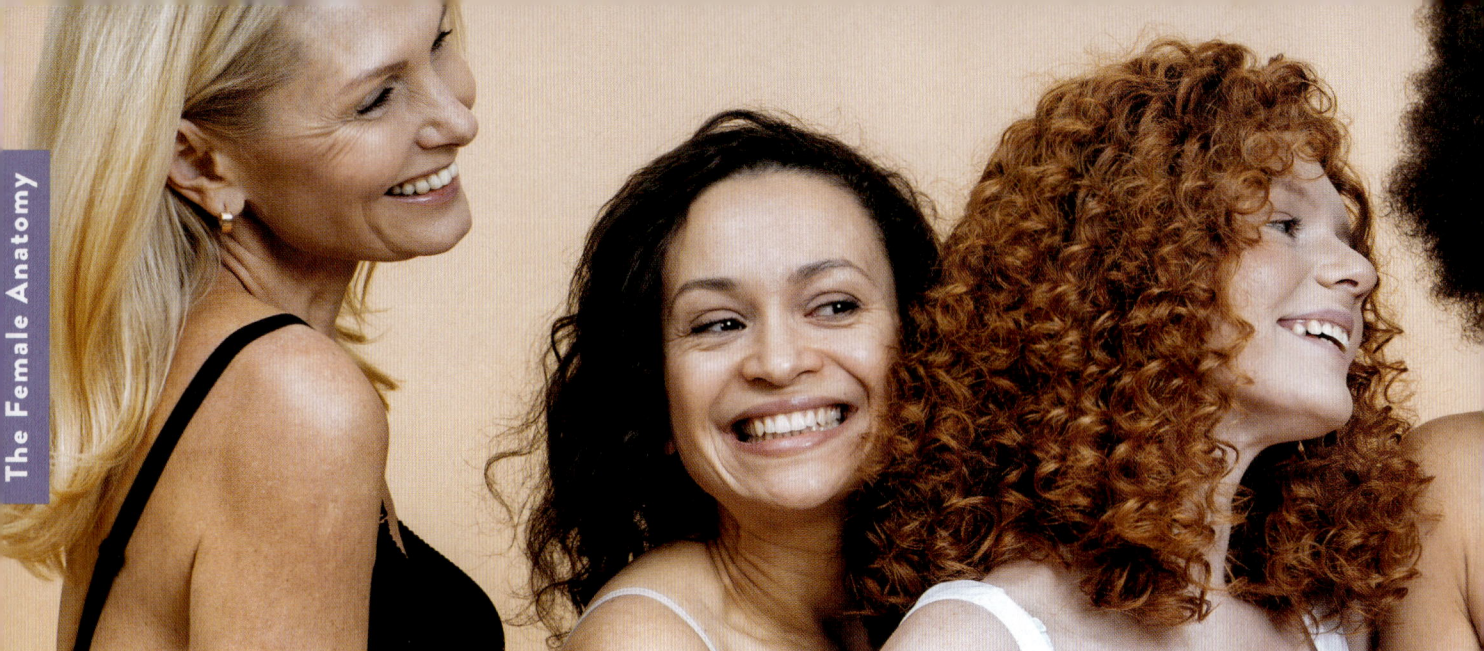

THE FEMALE
ANATOMY

Let's go back to basics! We explore female-specific body parts, both inside and out

While male and female human bodies have a lot in common, there are also key differences related to our sex that contribute to reproduction and hormone regulation, among other roles. You probably learned all about anatomy at school, but it never hurts to have a refresher.

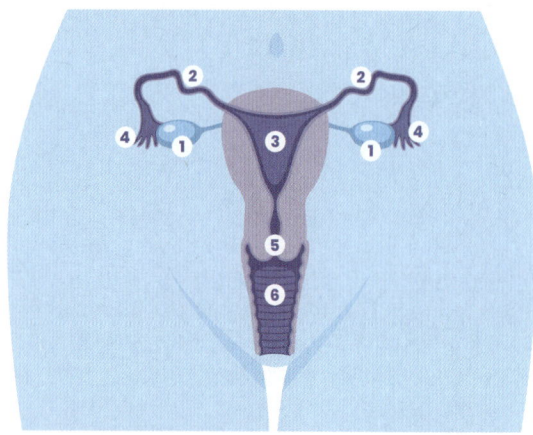

1. OVARIES
2. FALLOPIAN TUBES
3. UTERUS
4. FIMBRIAE
5. CERVIX
6. VAGINA

Understanding our anatomy can help us to become more aware of changes within our bodies, enabling us to keep track of our health. Female anatomy includes the internal and external parts of the reproductive system, the urinary system and the breasts. This short overview will also serve as a useful reference when we talk about specific parts of our anatomy throughout this guide.

The external parts of the reproductive and urinary systems form the vulva. The vulva includes the vaginal opening, which is surrounded by the labia majora and labia minor, both acting as protective skin layers. At the top of the vulva is the visible part of the clitoris (which stretches back into the body), and the urethral opening where urine is evacuated. Pubic hair typically grows on the mons pubis, a fatty area that sits on top of the pubic bone. There are also different glands found externally: the Bartholin's glands sit on both sides of the vaginal opening to help with lubrication, and the Skene's glands are on either side of the urethral opening and help to maintain urinary and sexual health.

The internal structure of the reproductive system is formed of numerous key parts. The vagina is the

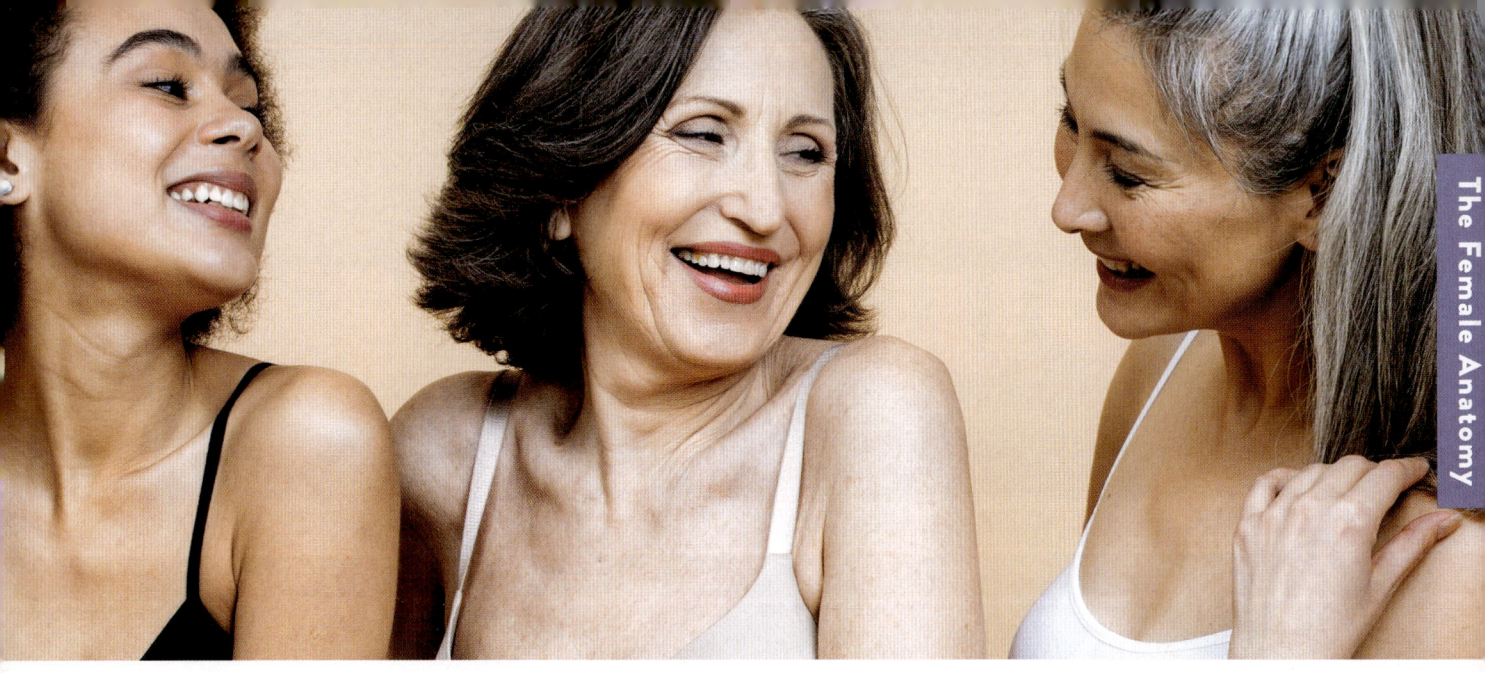

The Female Anatomy

1. **OVARY**
2. **FALLOPIAN TUBE**
3. **UTERUS**
4. **CERVIX**
5. **URINARY BLADDER**
6. **PUBIC BONE**
7. **VAGINA**
8. **CLITORIS**
9. **URETHRA**
10. **LABIUM MINORA**
11. **LABIUM MAJORA**
12. **ANUS**
13. **RECTUM**
14. **URETER**

> "UNDERSTANDING OUR ANATOMY HELPS US TO BE MORE AWARE OF CHANGES"

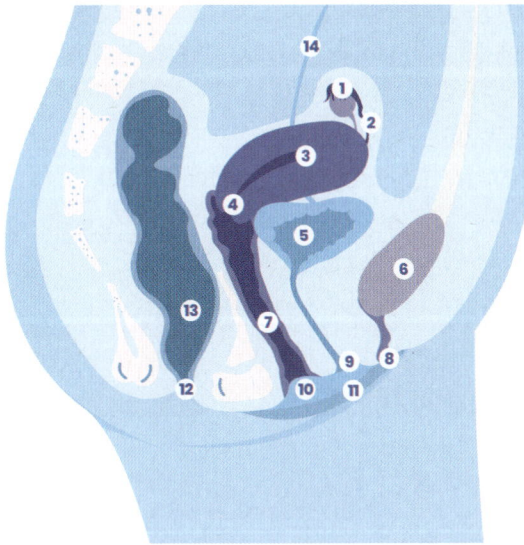

muscular canal that leads from the vaginal opening to the cervix, and it can contract and expand to enable sexual penetration and childbirth. The hymen is a thin piece of tissue that lies across the vaginal opening and will break at some point due to impact from exercise, sexual activity or one of many other causes. The cervix sits between the vagina and the uterus; during childbirth this dilates to enable the baby to move out of the uterus. The uterus (or womb) itself is part of the pelvic structure and is where a fertilised embryo develops into a foetus during pregnancy. Also within the pelvic area are the ovaries, which produce eggs and female sex hormones, and the fallopian tubes, which connect the ovaries with the uterus.

Female breasts have both an internal and external structure. Externally, there are the nipples at the centre of the breasts, and they can respond to stimulation or changes in temperature. Each nipple has milk duct openings to allow breast milk to flow through. The dark area around the nipple is called the areola, and this can change throughout your life in both size and colour, often triggered by hormonal changes or pregnancy.

Internally, breasts contain lobes, which have clusters of lobules responsible for producing breast milk. Milk ducts carry the milk produced by the lobules to the openings at the nipples. The breast also has blood vessels to carry nutrients and oxygen into the breast tissue, as well as lymph vessels connected to the lymph nodes in the armpits and chest that form part of the body's immune system. The breast itself is made up of fat tissue, called adipose, and this is what determines the size of the breast.

1. **PECTORAL MUSCLE**
2. **FAT CELLS**
3. **BLOOD VESSELS**
4. **LOBULES**
5. **NIPPLE**
6. **AREOLA**
7. **MILK DUCT**
8. **RIB**
9. **CHEST WALL**
10. **LUNG**

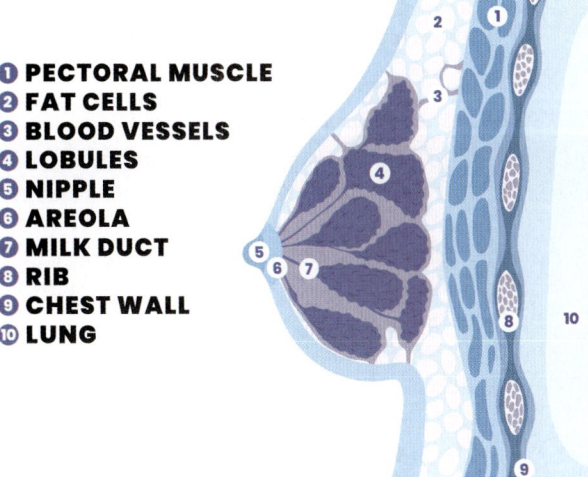

WHAT HAPPENS DURING PUBERTY?

The physical and psychological leaps that come with puberty and adolescence are pivotal to our body and health in adulthood

Throughout a woman's life, there are key developmental points associated with huge hormonal changes, which impact on both our physical and mental health. The first of these is around puberty and the adolescent years. In this feature, we explore what puberty actually is, what happens to our bodies around this time, and how this prepares us for becoming an adult.

Puberty is defined as the time when a child's body develops and matures into an adult body, in particular its reproductive capabilities. It is associated with reaching sexual maturity and gaining the ability to reproduce, though this is purely from a physiology point of view, as it can take a much longer time to reach emotional maturity. The term 'adolescence' refers to the period of time after the start of puberty up until reaching adulthood.

Puberty doesn't happen overnight, and every child develops at a different rate. There are huge changes happening in the brain and body during these adolescent years, which set us up for adulthood. For a girl, puberty usually begins any time between the ages of 8 and 14 years, though there are some cases where puberty is early or delayed (see the box below). ▶

> "EVERY CHILD DEVELOPS AT A DIFFERENT RATE"

EARLY & DELAYED PUBERTY

Sometimes young girls experience puberty outside the normal age range

The age at which puberty begins is quite variable, with wide parameters for what is considered 'normal'. However, it's possible for children to develop at a different time to their peers and outside of the usual age range. Early puberty, which is also called precocious puberty, is when girls exhibit signs of puberty before the age of eight (for boys it's before nine, though it's less common in boys). They may only experience one or two signs of puberty (such as starting periods), but it's always worth speaking to a doctor if a child does show these early indications. Early puberty can run in families, or it can be linked to underlying health problems or conditions. At the other end of the scale, delayed puberty is considered to be if a girl has not developed breasts by 13 years old, or they have developed breasts but not started their period by the age of 15. Again, this is something that can run in families, but it also should be checked out as there can be an underlying reason.

What Happens During Puberty?

DIFFERENCE IN SEXES
The average age for a girl to experience puberty is 11 years old. For boys the average age is 12 years old.

▶ BRAIN DEVELOPMENT

Puberty is a time of significant development in the brain. During adolescence, the brain undergoes remarkable changes in preparation for adulthood, with the brain usually fully mature by the time a person reaches their mid-20s. Most of these changes are internal, with different connections between parts of the brain being strengthened or pruned as needed. The physical brain is already at up to 95% of its adult size by age six, and fully grown by early adolescence. What is happening during puberty is that the brain is filtering what it needs and what it doesn't – connections that haven't been actively used are eliminated, making the brain more efficient, and new functions are being developed. This development happens over a long time, with different parts of the brain being developed at different speeds.

One area that develops in adolescence is the limbic system, which helps us to regulate our behaviour, emotions, motivation and memory function. The increase in activity in this area is responsible for the risk-taking and impulsivity that can occur in the teenage years. It can also mean heightened emotions and higher levels of stress. The other area that matures in adolescence is in the pre-frontal cortex, which is responsible for things like decision-making and reasoning, as well as being the centre of our personality traits. This is one of the last areas of the brain to finish developing; in the later teenage years and early adulthood, a young person becomes more able to think rationally, make better judgements, plan effectively and build healthy relationships.

These developments are shaped by our own experiences and environment, and no brain develops in the same way as another. It can be a challenging time both for young people and their caregivers – it can lead to a complete change in personality, behaviour and reasoning. However, the brain changes that occur during puberty and the experiences you have around this time are what make you who you are as an adult.

HORMONES IN PUBERTY

During puberty, our body starts to make more of certain hormones to signal to the body what changes are needed to develop towards adulthood. Puberty is controlled by a particular set of hormones found in the hypothalamic-pituitary-gonadal (HPG) axis. The hypothalamus is an

> **"THE BRAIN IS USUALLY FULLY MATURE BY THE TIME A PERSON REACHES THEIR MID-20s"**

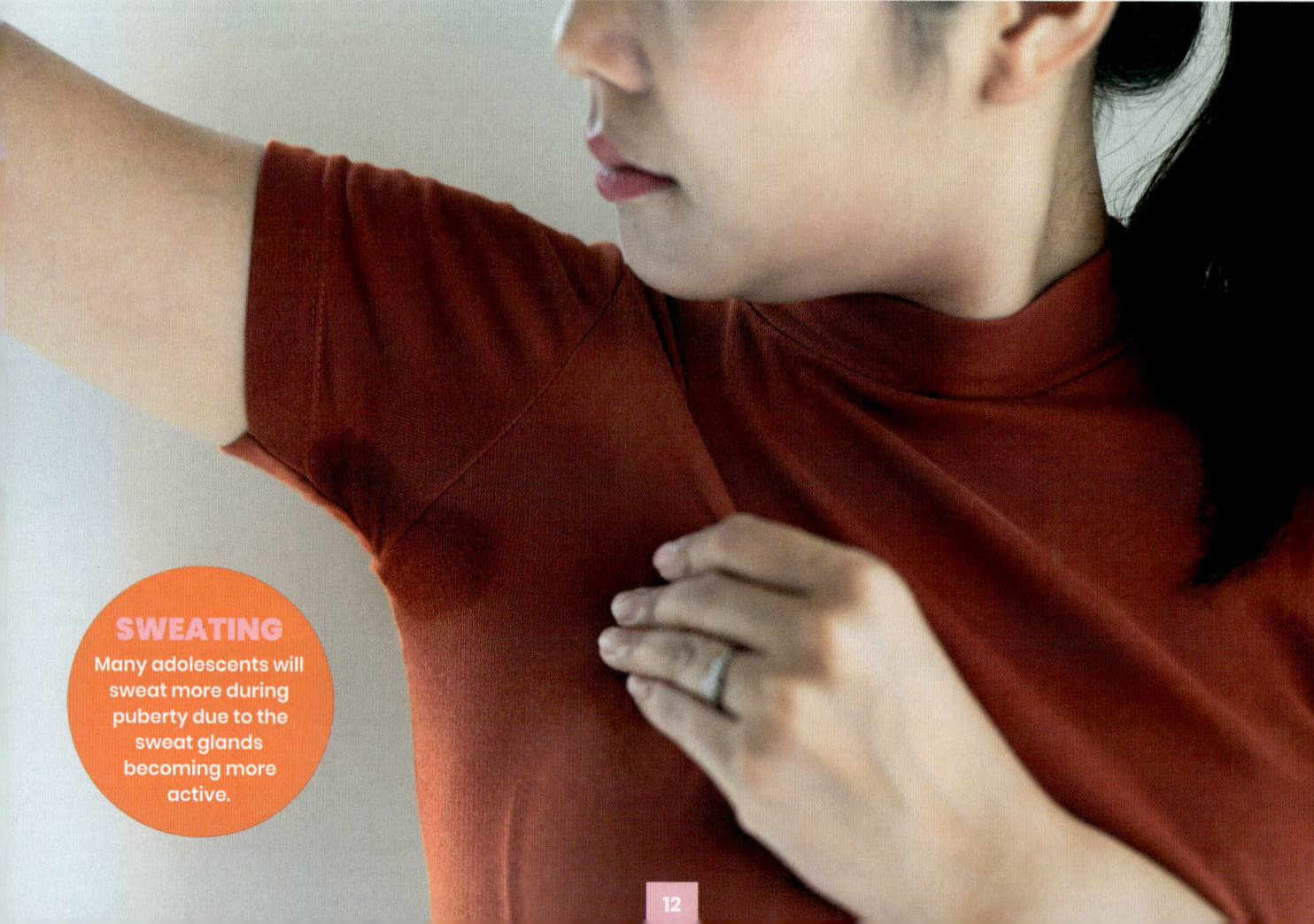

SWEATING
Many adolescents will sweat more during puberty due to the sweat glands becoming more active.

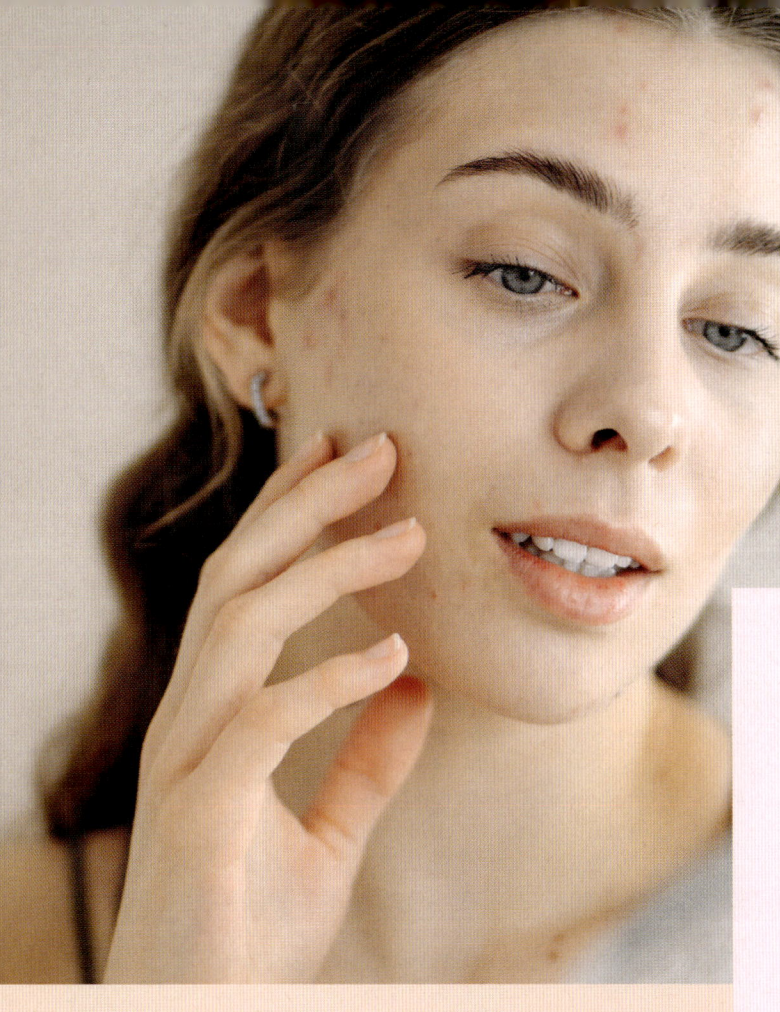

What Happens During Puberty?

ACNE IN PUBERTY & BEYOND

Many people experience problems with their skin during the adolescent years

We've already explained how hormones are released in greater quantities during puberty, including testosterone. This triggers an increase in the production of sebum, an oily substance that's produced by the sebaceous glands. An excess in sebum can lead to acne, a skin complaint that is often associated with teenagers. It's so common that 85% of 16 to 18-year-olds can be affected.[2] Usually, acne improves from about the age of 25. However, you might continue to experience acne into adulthood for various reasons, including certain medications or cosmetics, environmental conditions, diet, or an underlying medical cause such as polycystic ovary syndrome. Some women also find that they struggle with acne during perimenopause as their hormones begin to fluctuate. It's more common for women to experience adult acne than men, and flare-ups can be linked to the patterns of the menstrual cycle. Adult acne can require different treatment than teenage acne, so it's also worth consulting with a dermatologist for advice.

important part of the brain, controlling body temperature, hunger and thirst cues, mood, sex drive and sleep. As the brain matures, the hypothalamus releases something called gonadotropin releasing hormone (GnRH), which in turn triggers the release of key hormones that kickstart puberty.

Luteinising hormone (LH) and follicle-stimulating hormone (FSH) are produced by the pituitary gland – which is an important gland that helps to control things like blood pressure, energy levels and thyroid function, among other things. LH and FSH together are what tell the ovaries to produce more oestrogen and progesterone. LH and FSH levels are typically high in a newborn baby, but they fall and stay low throughout childhood. Measuring these hormone levels is one way of determining if a child is going into puberty early.

In girls, there is then a marked increase in the production of female sex hormones, primarily oestrogen and progesterone. FSH is what triggers the increase in oestrogen, and LH stimulates the production of progesterone. Girls also start to produce more testosterone than they did pre-puberty, with levels higher in later puberty. Together, these key hormones prepare the reproductive capabilities of the body and are responsible for the physical changes that occur.

PHYSICAL CHANGES

Due to these hormonal changes, a young girl's body will begin to change in response. It's not ▶

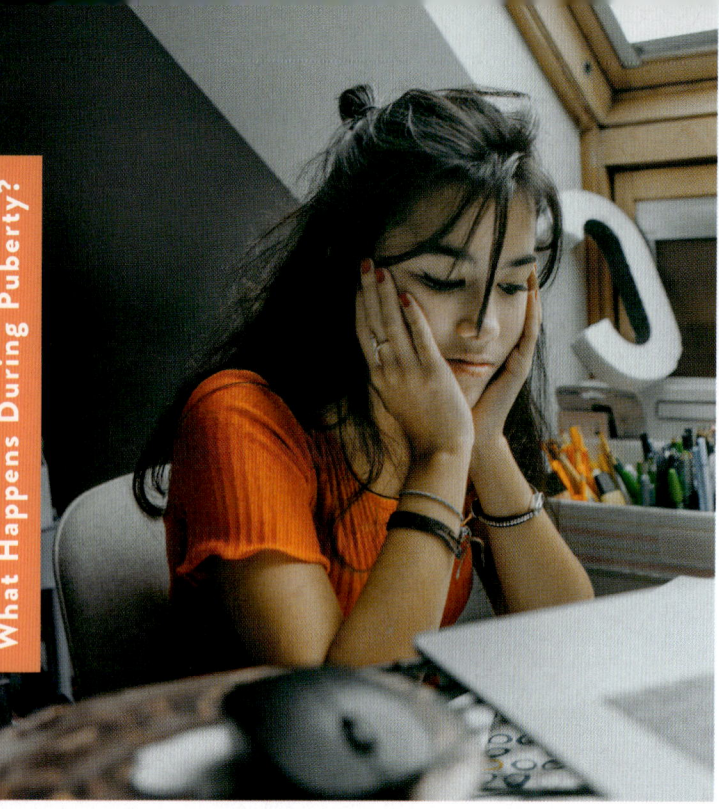

FINISHING PUBERTY

While it might not feel like it at the time, puberty does come to an end

There is an end point to puberty, when the body and brain have finished their developments, and a young girl has become an adult woman. For most girls, puberty itself ends any time between the ages of 15 to 16, but just as with the way it starts, there is huge variation. Puberty normally lasts for around five to six years, so for those who begin puberty a little later, it may carry on longer too. At this point, the body will stop making significant physical changes. A person usually reaches their final adult height before the age of 18, for example, and the reproductive system reaches full maturity. Hormones levels also begin to stabilise again, and the menstrual cycle may become more regular and predictable. A young adult may also have more stable emotions, better resilience and balanced moods, as well as a better sense of who they are.

unusual for a girl to have a growth spurt around this time – normally earlier than boys do, so they may often be the taller sex in the early adolescent years. The biggest spurt in height can often occur around the same time that breast buds appear and before periods begin. Once periods have been established, growth tends to slow down.

One of the first signs of puberty is often the development of breast buds, which feel like small coin-sized bumps underneath the nipple. They may feel a little sore or itchy, and they will continue to grow over time. This can often happen much earlier than parents expect – from as young as eight years old. The buds may also develop unevenly, but in most cases will even out over time. As they get bigger, it's often time to think about training bras. It's also a good idea to have discussions around breast health so that young girls are comfortable with learning what looks and feels normal. This can go towards creating a habit of regular breast checks in adulthood to help detect any problems early. Breasts are normally fully developed by the late teenage years, though they will change in appearance and size throughout a person's life. The breasts develop under the skin too. The increase in oestrogen helps to build the duct system, and progesterone increases the number of lobules. Once a menstrual cycle has been established, increased fat deposits in the area start to build up the breast shape.

The formation of breast buds is often followed by the first signs of pubic hair, although in some cases hair growth can occur first. This is followed by underarm air and leg hair as a child moves further into puberty, and they may become curious about shaving. Hair may also become a little greasier at this time, and many young girls struggle with skin issues, such as spots and acne.

> **"FOR MOST GIRLS, PUBERTY ENDS BETWEEN THE AGES OF 15 TO 16"**

The most obvious, and sometimes worrying, development for any girl going through puberty is their first period. This happens about two years after the initial breast buds appear – though the timeline is different for every child. The average age for starting periods is around 12 years old, but again there is a lot of variation. There are many factors that can dictate the onset of menstruation, including body weight, environment, genetics, race and ethnicity (Black girls, for example, are more likely to start puberty a little earlier).[1]

The female body changes shape during puberty. This includes a widening of the hips in preparation for childbirth in later life, and an increase in body fat. However, the body composition also changes, so early childhood fat ('puppy fat') around the waist may disappear, with any increase in body fat accumulating more around the hips and thighs, creating a different shape.

Other physical changes happen in puberty in the reproductive organs. The vagina and vulva grow bigger, and the uterus also increases in size in preparation for the potential to host a baby. The ovaries will become more mature and ready to start releasing eggs, triggering the start of a menstrual cycle. Around this time, vaginal discharge may start to appear to help keep the area healthy, which is usually clear or white.

EMOTIONAL CHANGES

As well as the physical effects that occur in puberty, it's a time when a young person goes through a lot of emotional and psychological changes. The combination of hormones rushing in and the development of the brain can lead to mood and behaviour changes, as well as feelings of stress and being overwhelmed. It's not uncommon to experience mood swings, often going from one extreme to another in a matter of minutes. It's hard to understand what's going on when you're going through it, but it's part of the process of growing up and discovering a deeper set of emotions and thought processes. The emotional resilience that we learn in adolescence equips us to deal better with the stresses of adult life.

Puberty can also be a time when pre-teens and teenagers try to figure out who they are, and these discoveries can inform the kind of adults we become. These years are often when young people start to explore relationships more and look at their own friendship groups in a different light. This can lead to changing dynamics within peer groups, which can often be a cause of stress and upset, but it's a normal part of finding their own way in the world. Adolescents may also become more self-conscious, particularly if their body has changed a lot, and they may become more sensitive to different emotions and triggers.

With a growing, but not yet developed, ability to self-regulate, it's no wonder that mental health problems can crop up more frequently in the early teenage years. According to the Mental Health Foundation, 20% of adolescents may experience a mental-health problem in any given year, and 50% of mental-health problems are established by age 14 (75% by age 24). If you're a parent or caregiver for a young person, keep an eye on signs that they may be struggling with their mental health and seek help if you're worried. If you have mental-health problems in adulthood, it's possible that you can identify a trigger based on your own adolescent years.

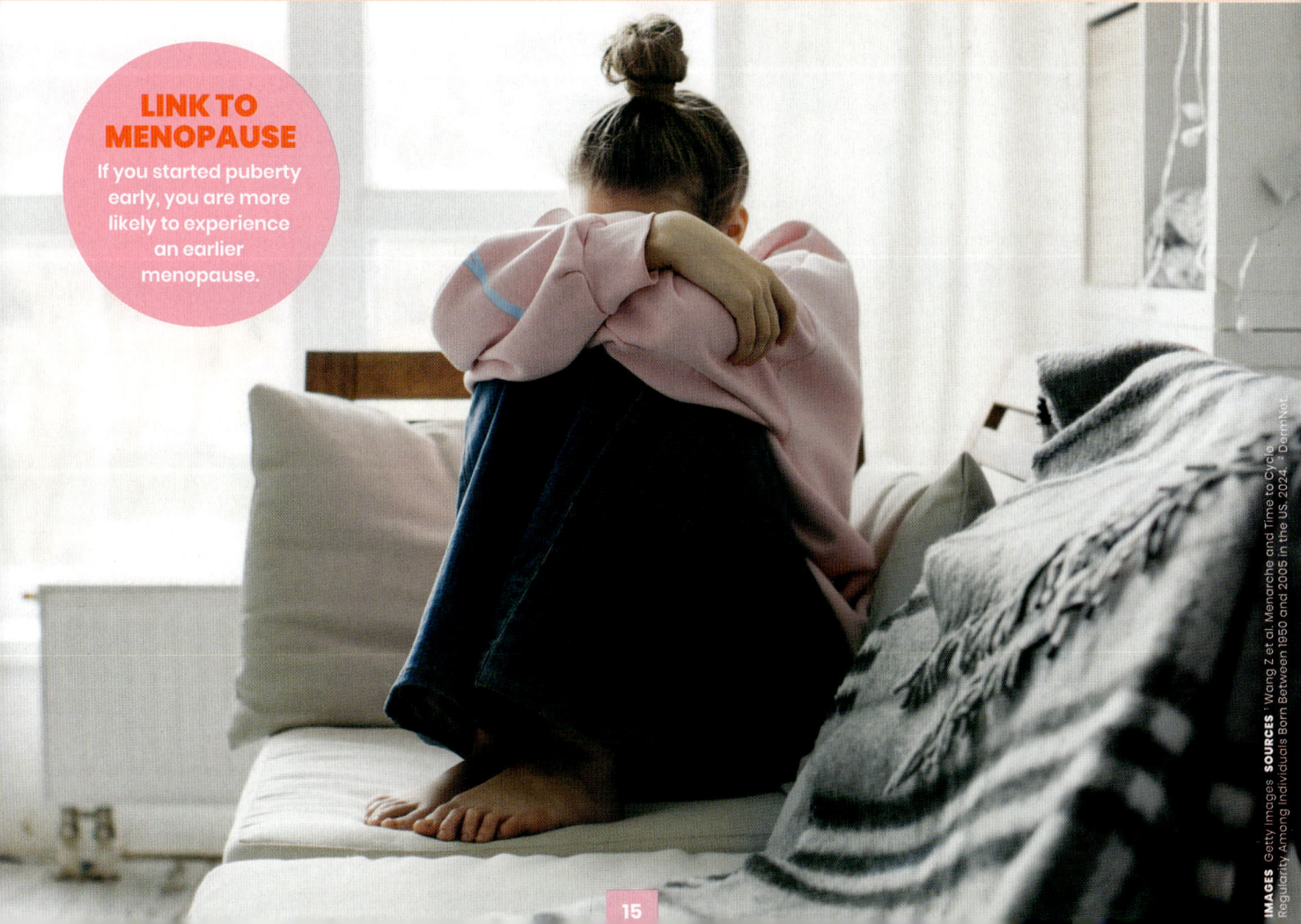

LINK TO MENOPAUSE
If you started puberty early, you are more likely to experience an earlier menopause.

A Guide To Essential Hormones

COMMON ISSUES
It's thought that up to 80% of women have some form of hormonal imbalance.

A GUIDE TO ESSENTIAL HORMONES

Your hormones play an important role throughout your life; let's take a look at the ones that have the most impact

Hormones are a type of chemical molecule in the body that carry messages to organs and tissues to enable them to carry out their functions. We often focus on the sex hormones, as they can have the biggest impact on our overall health and wellness, but there are more than 50 different hormones that keep our body working optimally. All our hormones should, ideally, be in balance, which enables us to be in good health, but having a hormonal imbalance is not unusual. Identifying which hormones need treatment, however, can be more complex, as the symptoms of a hormonal imbalance can be very general (see the box on the following page).

Hormones are produced by glands situated all over the body. This network of glands is called the endocrine system, and it works alongside the nervous system, immune system and respiratory system. The endocrine system can be disrupted by external influences, such as coming into contact with certain chemicals in food or our environment. When the body produces too few or too many hormones it can lead to health complications.

FEMALE HORMONES

Within the female body there are two main groups of hormones that are responsible for reproductive capabilities, and these can have a noticeable effect on our health. The first is oestrogen (or estrogen, which is another common spelling), of which there are numerous types. We tend to just group them all under the umbrella term of 'oestrogen', but the three main individual hormones are oestrone, oestradiol and oestriol. Together their main function is to develop secondary sex characteristics (such as breasts), maintain the menstrual cycle and support pregnancy. But they do a lot more than that; oestrogen also helps to support your brain, bones, skin and heart, which is why these are such a critical set of hormones.

Each of the individual hormone types contribute to your health in different ways and at different times of your life. Oestrone is mainly produced by the ovaries, as well as by fat tissue and the adrenal glands. It's generally less active as a hormone in your earlier years, but post-menopause, when the ovaries stop producing as many hormones, oestrone becomes the primary source of oestrogen. The dominant type of oestrogen is oestradiol, which is the key hormone when it comes to maintaining reproductive capabilities. It is what enables us to mature an egg to be released during ovulation, but it also helps to support bone health. Finally, oestriol is more related to pregnancy. It is present in relatively low levels most of the time, but levels increase during pregnancy, peaking just before birth. It helps the uterus to expand and prepare for labour. ▶

> "THERE ARE MORE THAN 50 DIFFERENT HORMONES THAT KEEP OUR BODY WORKING OPTIMALLY"

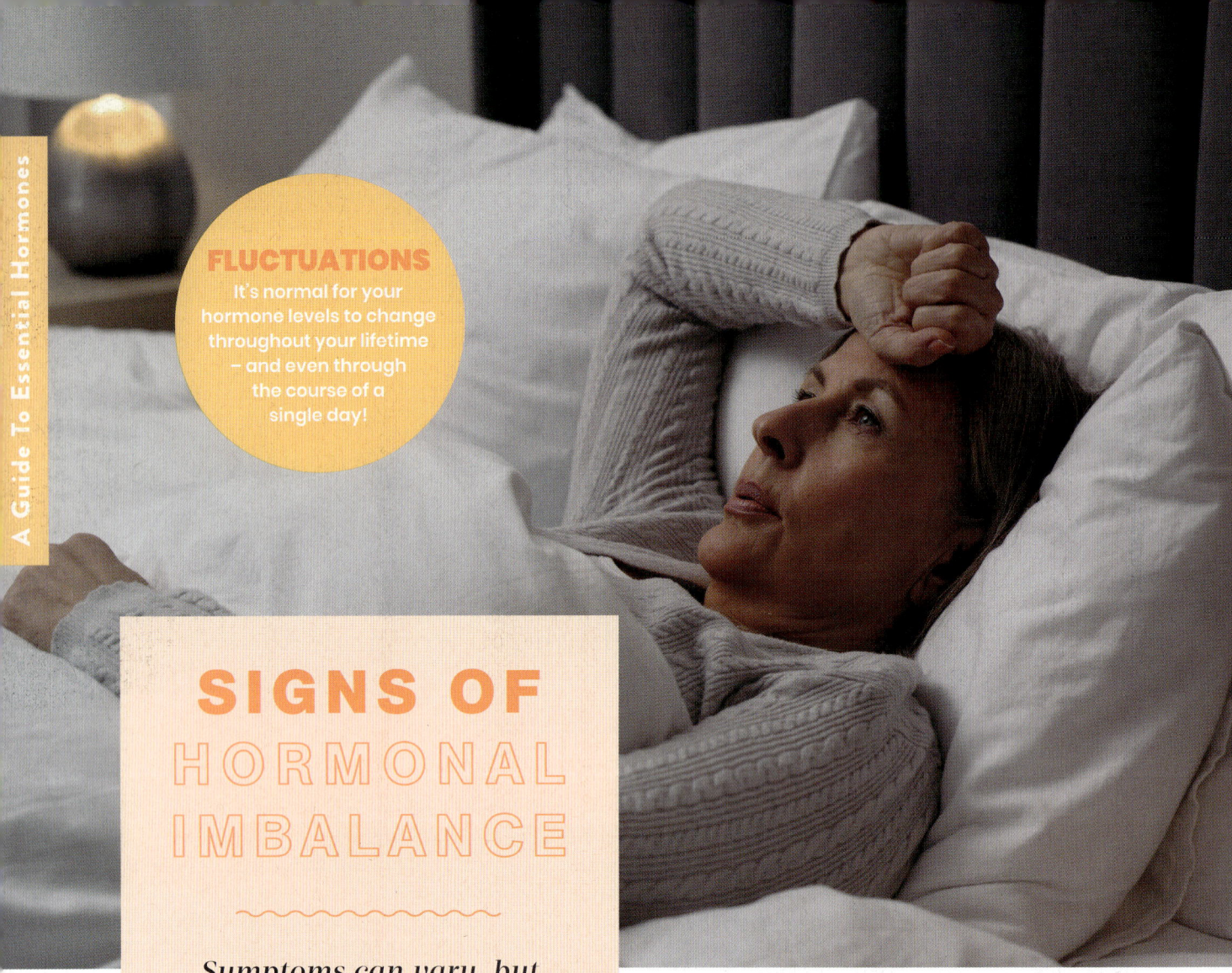

FLUCTUATIONS
It's normal for your hormone levels to change throughout your lifetime – and even through the course of a single day!

SIGNS OF HORMONAL IMBALANCE

Symptoms can vary, but there are signs you shouldn't ignore

Hormonal imbalances can leave you feeling off, but many of the key symptoms can also be symptoms of lots of different conditions. That's why if you feel like something isn't right, it's worth speaking to a doctor to get some tests to eliminate or discover the underlying reason for the way you're feeling. Things to watch out for include any changes to your general mood – such as the onset of, or increase in, anxiety or depression – or noticeable mood swings. You may also notice a lower sex drive than normal, weight gain or weight loss, dry skin or hair, changes to your menstrual cycle, problems with sleep, acne, headaches, changes to heart rate, increased fatigue or digestive issues. Given the breadth of symptoms, hormonal imbalances have the potential to impact lots of areas of your life. It's also worth bearing in mind that many of these symptoms can be associated with the start of perimenopause.

▶ The other key female sex hormone is progesterone, which also helps to regulate the menstrual cycle and support pregnancy. Alongside this are luteinising hormone (LH) and follicle-stimulating hormone (FSH), which both contribute to a healthy menstrual cycle. Over the course of a menstrual cycle, the female hormones ebb and flow to support the body at different stages. During your period, levels of oestrogen and progesterone are low. In the lead up to ovulation, the body starts to produce more FSH, which stimulates the ovaries to create follicles containing immature eggs, which in turn releases more oestrogen. As oestrogen levels continue to rise, this triggers the release of LH to begin ovulation and release a mature egg. When the egg is released, progesterone levels increase to help thicken the lining of the uterus in preparation for the possibility of pregnancy. If you get pregnant, another hormone called human chorionic gonadotropin (hCG) is produced to help keep the uterus healthy, and this is the hormone that pregnancy tests can detect. If no fertilisation takes place, then your body will shed the thickened uterine lining and your hormone levels will drop again, ready to begin a new menstrual cycle.

If you do get pregnant, the body will create more of the hormone prolactin, which helps with breast milk production. Prolactin does have other roles

THE ENDOCRINE SYSTEM

Key hormones are produced throughout your body – this diagram shows the primary locations

1 PINEAL GLAND
Produces melatonin to help regulate sleep cycles

2 HYPOTHALAMUS
Helps regulate body temperature, appetite, weight, mood, sleep and thirst

3 PITUITARY GLAND
Produces hormones that support growth, reproduction and lactation

4 THYROID GLAND
Helps to control metabolism and heart function

5 THYMUS
Helps to fight infection, as part of the immune system

6 PANCREAS
Produces insulin to help control blood sugar levels

7 ADRENAL GLANDS
Produce androgens and cortisol, regulating stress and blood pressure

8 OVARIES
Produce the female sex hormones, including oestrogen and progesterone

> "WHEN YOU'RE UNDER STRESS, CORTISOL TRIGGERS YOUR BODY'S DEFENCE SYSTEM"

within the body as well, including breast tissue development, sex drive and bone health. Testosterone is thought of as a male sex hormone, and while it is the primary hormone in men, it is important for women too. Small amounts of testosterone are produced in the ovaries, helping with muscle and bone health, as well as libido.

The female sex hormones change throughout our lives and are associated with big periods of change. In our section on puberty and adolescence we explain how hormone levels begin to rise. The body starts to produce more oestrogen, triggering puberty and changing our bodies in preparation for adulthood. During the reproductive years, oestrogen and progesterone stabilise, rising and dropping throughout a menstrual cycle in a regular (or irregular) cycle. As we get older and approach menopause, these hormones start to fluctuate, causing all manner of symptoms, which we'll explore later on. Eventually, the level of hormones will drop low enough to cease reproductive abilities for good. Post-menopause, hormone levels remain low but stable.

ADRENAL HORMONES

At the top of both of your kidneys are the adrenal glands, which produce key hormones that impact on your general health. You may have heard of cortisol, which is often referred to as the 'stress hormone' due to the role it plays in helping to manage your response to stress. When we are in a stressful situation, cortisol is released. This is a natural response to stress, but having too much cortisol over a long time (chronic stress) can cause symptoms. When you're under stress, cortisol triggers your body's own defence system. This includes the release of adrenaline so that you're on alert to respond to the stress, as well as stimulating the release of glucose from the liver to help give you a surge of energy to fight the perceived threat. But cortisol isn't just needed for this 'fight or flight' response. It's an important part of your metabolism, helping to regulate your energy levels. It also helps to control inflammation, regulate blood pressure and maintain a healthy sleep cycle. If you are ▶

A Guide To Essential Hormones

HORMONE REPLACEMENT THERAPY
HRT replaces the oestrogen and progesterone that decline naturally in menopause, helping to relieve symptoms.

THYROID PROBLEMS

Around one in eight women will develop a problem with their thyroid over their lifetime[1]

The thyroid gland is an important part of the endocrine system, producing key hormones that are essential to regulate your metabolism. The most common thyroid issue is when it doesn't produce enough hormones – this is known as an underactive thyroid, or hypothyroidism. There's no way to prevent it from happening; the most common cause is an autoimmune condition called Hashimoto's disease, where the immune system attacks the thyroid gland. Other causes of an underactive thyroid can include treatment for thyroid cancer or an overactive thyroid, which can damage the thyroid gland. The symptoms of an underactive thyroid include more tiredness than usual, unexplained weight gain, feeling low or depressed, dry skin and hair, muscle aches, and sensitivity to cold. These symptoms can also be linked to other conditions, so the only way to diagnose is to have a thyroid function test.

It's also possible to have an overactive thyroid, or hyperthyroidism, which is when the gland produces too many hormones. It typically affects women (10 times more so than men) aged between 20 and 40. Symptoms include anxiety, irritability, mood swings, problems sleeping, tiredness, sensitivity to heat, heart palpitations and weight loss. It's also possible for the thyroid gland to swell, causing a lump called a goitre.

pregnant, cortisol also helps to support a developing foetus.

Adrenaline is produced in the adrenal glands. It causes more oxygen to flow into the muscles and more blood to pass to the major organs. It also decreases the pain response, and can lead to a temporary strength boost and heightened awareness. All of these are part of a system to survive against dangers, though adrenaline can be released when there isn't any real danger, but the brain perceives a threat. Adrenaline works alongside the hormone norepinephrine, also produced in the adrenal glands, which increases heart rate, blood flow and blood sugar. Outside of a stress situation, norepinephrine plays an important role in our sleep cycles and emotional health.

CONTROL CENTRE OF THE BRAIN

There are two key areas in the brain that release hormones essential to our health and wellbeing. The pituitary gland is a small, pea-sized gland located at the base of the brain under the hypothalamus. As well as releasing important hormones itself, it also helps to control the release of hormones from other glands throughout the body. The pituitary gland produces the aforementioned FSH, LH and prolactin hormones that are an important part of the reproductive cycle. It produces growth hormones that help us grow taller, and build healthy muscles and bones, and aids metabolism. It also produces ACTH, a hormone that triggers the release of cortisol from the adrenal glands when under stress. The pituitary gland is responsible for stimulating the thyroid gland to produce hormones (see the box on the previous page on thyroid problems).

The hypothalamus is often called the control centre of the brain, because of its role in maintaining your body and health. It acts as the link between your endocrine system and your nervous system, sending instructions to both to keep you in a stable state. It receives and sends messages throughout your body and triggers the appropriate responses. This includes managing things like your body temperature, your blood pressure, your appetite and thirst, your mood, your sex drive and your sleep-wake cycle. It also makes some hormones directly, even if they are released from other parts of your body. It works alongside the pituitary gland to ensure your endocrine system is working as it should.

Some of the hormones that come from the hypothalamus include oxytocin, which supports with childbirth and lactation among other things; and vasopressin, which helps to control your urine levels and blood pressure. It also produces dopamine, which helps to give us a sense of pleasure and motivation. Dopamine levels are increased during exercise or when we're doing something we enjoy.

OTHER HORMONES

The pancreas produces important hormones that help to regulate our blood sugar levels. There are two main hormones that impact on this. Glucagon helps to control our glucose levels, preventing them from dropping too low. It works together in balance with insulin, one of the most important hormones in our body, which is responsible for lowering blood sugar levels. It is pivotal for turning the food we eat into energy that we can use and moving it into the body's cells. The body also stores glucose for future use as glycogen, which can be released for energy when we need it. If your body doesn't produce enough insulin, or doesn't use it effectively, glucose can't get out of your bloodstream and into the cells, which leads to high blood sugar levels and diabetes. Diabetes can sometimes be managed by injecting insulin to help reduce these levels.

Other hormones that you may have heard of include melatonin, which is a hormone that regulates the sleep-wake cycle. It is produced in the brain, rising at night to help you rest and lowering in the day to keep you alert. Serotonin acts as a hormone that regulates your mood and appetite, among other functions. Low serotonin levels can contribute to mental-health conditions like depression or anxiety. Leptin helps us to regulate appetite and maintain a healthy weight, and GLP-1 is produced by the gut after eating to aid with appetite and digestion.

There are many other hormones that operate in the body, but we've given you an overview of the main ones that might impact you day to day. Hopefully this has given you a better understanding of the delicate balance of your endocrine system.

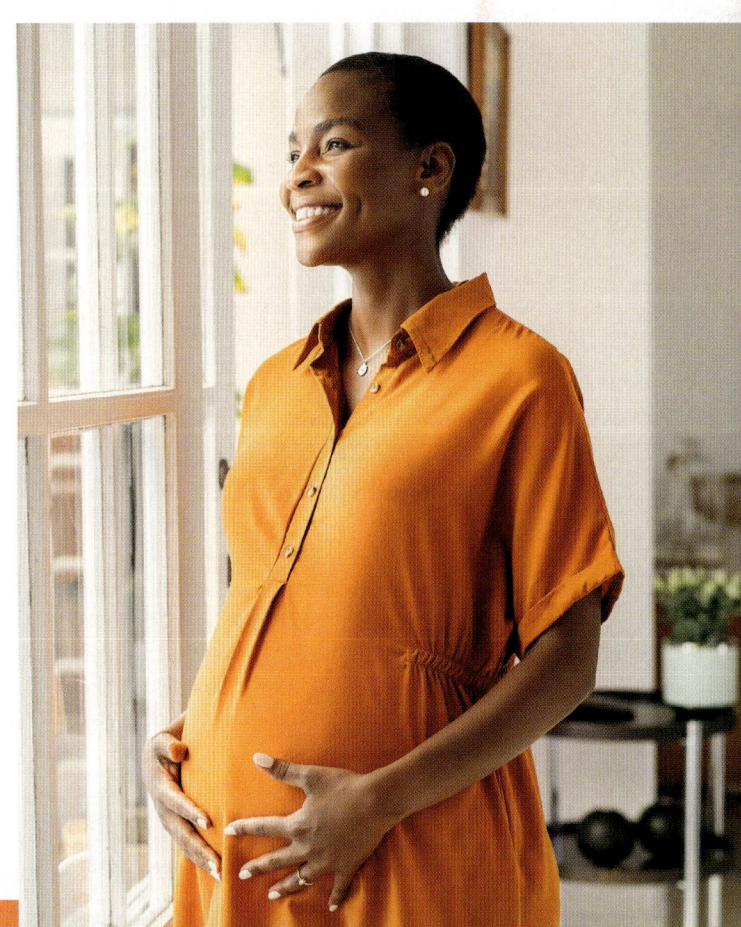

IMAGES Getty Images SOURCES ¹Office on Women's Health, US government

WHAT IS GOOD HEALTH?

We always talk about being 'fit and healthy', but what does that mean and how does it make us feel?

What does 'being healthy' mean to you? Chances are that we would all give different answers to that question, as feeling healthy in ourselves depends on our outcomes and the environment we live in and are exposed to. For example, if you spend time on social media, you might see one specific definition of health – a particular diet, a certain body type, the 'right' type of exercise to do. And then you might follow that advice and find yourself feeling run down, burned out or unable to meet your expectations – does that really sound healthy?

On one hand, you might have a person who follows a strict diet and exercises daily, but has multiple medical conditions. And on the other you could have someone who smokes, is overweight and drinks alcohol, but has a completely clean bill of health. Or maybe a person is doing really well on metrics like diet and exercise, but suffers with anxiety and depression. Which of these people is healthy?

This shows that it's not just about one thing or another, and having good health is a combination of a balanced lifestyle, feeling physically, mentally and socially well, as well as being at low risk of serious physical and mental-health conditions.

Some of us may already have underlying health issues, but that doesn't mean that it's not possible to be in good health – there are always challenges and obstacles that are personal to us, and what healthy looks like can vary hugely.

Let's have a look in more detail about how you can assess whether you're in good health, as well as the different areas of health to focus on. Throughout the next section of this book, we'll be looking in more detail at health conditions, diet and exercise, to help you work on the areas you identify as being those you need to work on the most.

SIGNS OF GOOD HEALTH

There are signs that indicate when you're in generally good health, and these are your body's way of telling you when something is working… and when it isn't. It's unlikely that you'll tick all the boxes, but by being aware of these signs, they can help you to figure out any improvements you need to make to work towards optimal health. Some of the metrics may not be possible for you to achieve due to underlying issues, but that's okay – we can all only do what we can, and every step is better than no step at all.

As a woman, one of the best signs of good health is having a regular menstrual cycle. Your body can only achieve this when you're in good health, your hormones are balanced and there are no medical issues. It means that the body isn't under too much stress (whether that's mental stress or physical, such as overtraining) and it's able to maintain its reproductive abilities. For women on hormonal contraception, however, this isn't a good metric, as the hormone intake disrupts the natural rhythms of the body. ▶

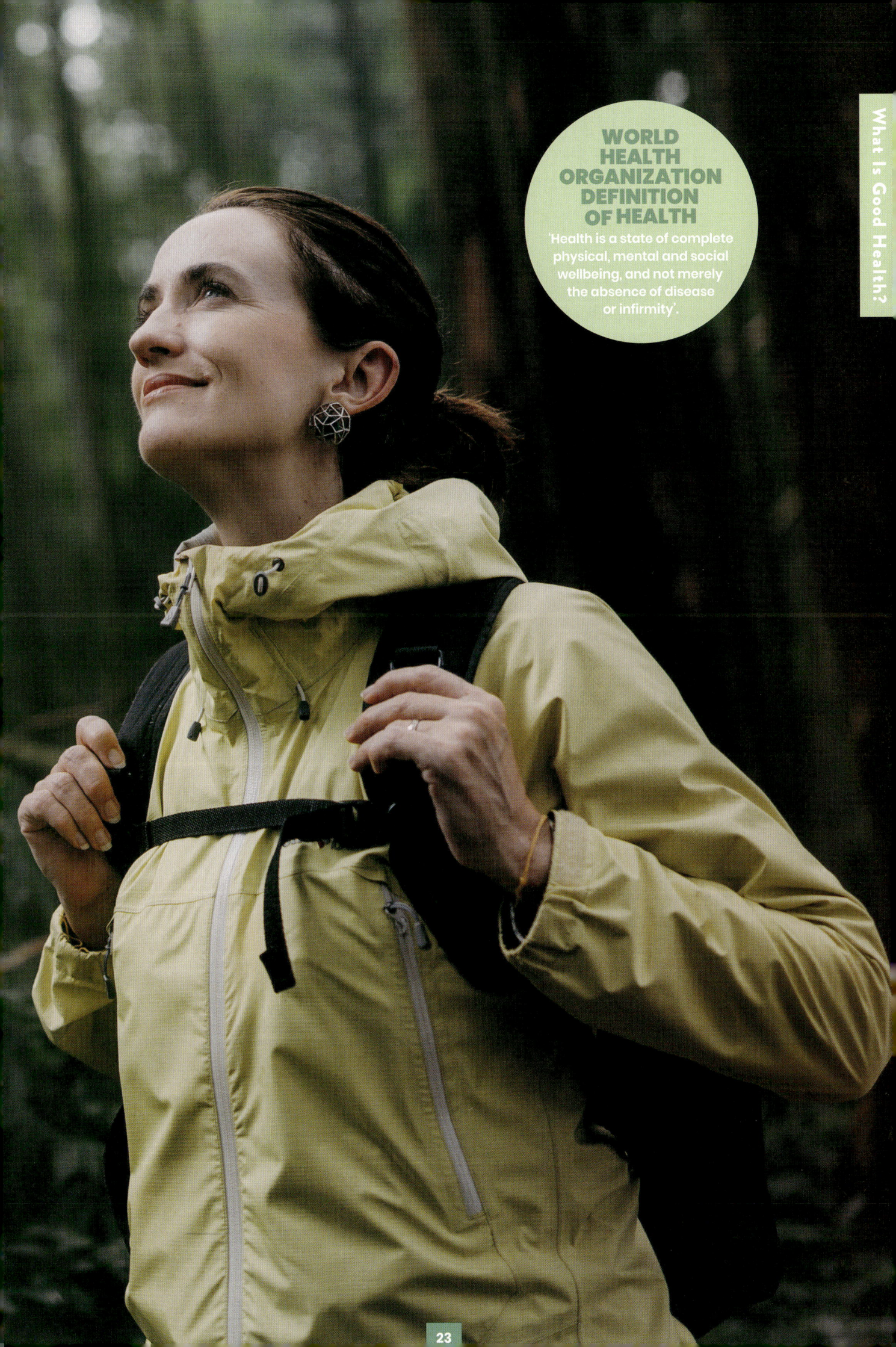

WORLD HEALTH ORGANIZATION DEFINITION OF HEALTH

'Health is a state of complete physical, mental and social wellbeing, and not merely the absence of disease or infirmity'.

What Is Good Health?

GOOD MENTAL HEALTH

Your mental wellbeing is just as important as your physical

There are also signs of good mental health, just as there are physical health indicators. If you're feeling mentally well, then you are more able to cope with life and any obstacles that come up. You probably feel generally more optimistic – or at least not pessimistic – as well as contented with your life. Good mental health brings about a sense of calmness and positivity, and can make it easier to maintain good relationships, connections and values. Being able to talk about your mental health is also a good sign. Those with good mental health are also more productive, focused and adaptable. It's normal to feel sadness, grief and anger in response to certain situations, but good mental health is about our resilience in these times and being able to maintain perspective. Your mental health will go up and down throughout your life, responding to different triggers, so it's also about being aware of any changes – and seeking support if you ever feel that your mental health is declining.

▶ Also, for those who may be approaching perimenopause and menopause, irregular periods are a normal part of the process. And monitoring your menstrual cycle as a sign of good health is not relevant for those who do not have periods due to health conditions or surgery.

Another sign of good health is whether you're getting enough consistent high-quality sleep. Sleep is a key process that enables our body to repair and restore itself, and not getting enough can impact on so many other areas of our wellbeing. You know when you're having good sleep if you fall asleep easily at night, don't wake in the night (or if you do wake, you get back to sleep easily) and you wake up feeling energised. Lack of sleep is linked to many physical and mental health problems.

> "SLEEP IS A KEY PROCESS THAT ENABLES OUR BODY TO REPAIR ITSELF"

Monitoring your energy levels can also indicate whether you're in good health. You should, ideally, have consistent and stable energy throughout the whole day, rather than peaks and troughs. This should mean that you're able to go about your daily activities and exercise without it affecting your energy too badly. If you're having to top up your energy levels with caffeine, for example, feeling that you need to have a nap or experience a mid-afternoon slump, then there may be areas of your health that need to be addressed. There are conditions that impact on energy levels too.

Toileting habits are always a good indicator of health, even if it's not something you feel inclined to check too often! Your bowel movements, in particular, are a good sign that your body is working optimally. You should be going to the toilet regularly and comfortably – check out the Bristol Stool Chart online to see what's normal. Similarly, you want a healthy urinary system, which is when you have pale-yellow urine that is passed without pain, regularly and without leakage.

Your skin, hair and nails will reflect your health too. Well hydrated, healthy and clear skin is a good sign of a well-functioning body. Things like dryness, itching, tightness or burning can indicate that there's something going on. Nails should also be nicely pink and well nourished, and your hair shiny and in good condition, with minimal hair loss or breakage. Your gums would ordinarily be a pink colour with minimal or no bleeding when brushing or flossing.

There are indicators inside your body too. Things like your heart rate, blood pressure, blood sugar levels, cholesterol and so on should all be within

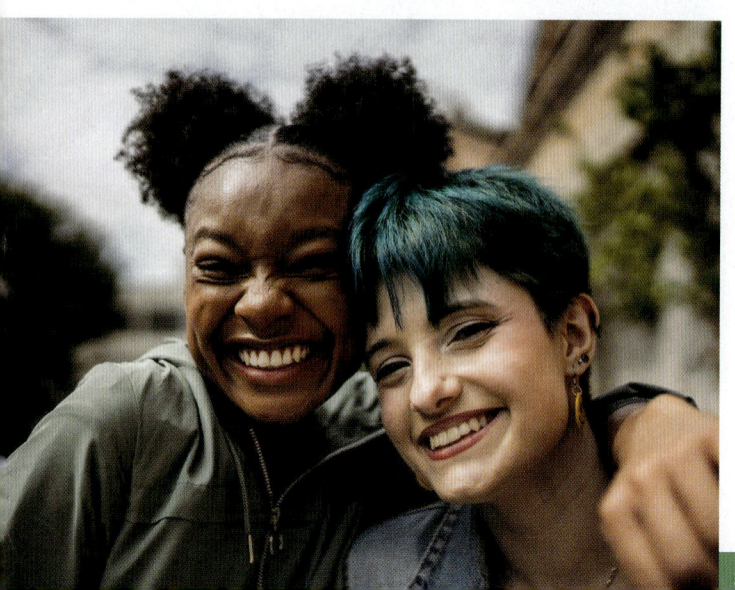

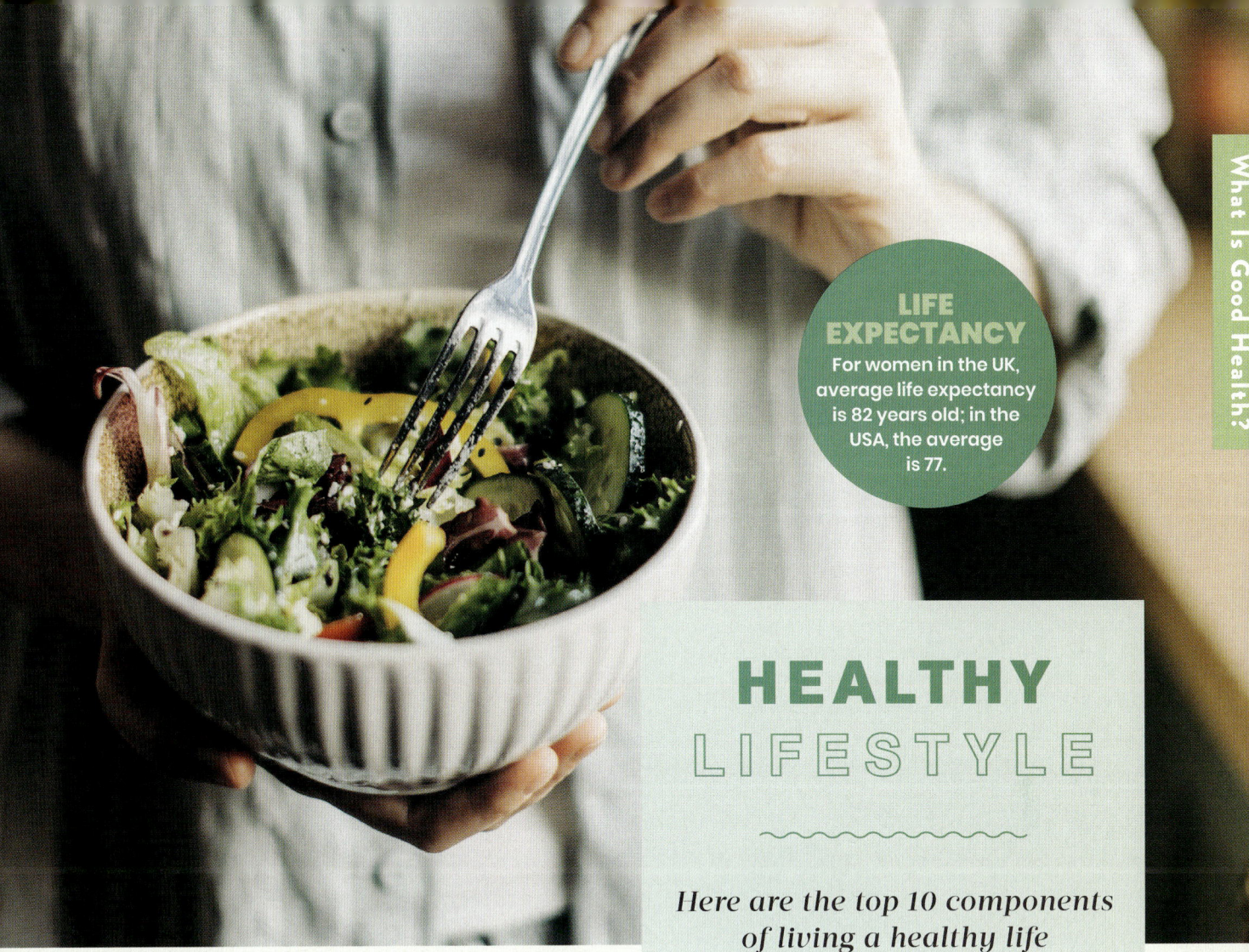

LIFE EXPECTANCY
For women in the UK, average life expectancy is 82 years old; in the USA, the average is 77.

HEALTHY LIFESTYLE

Here are the top 10 components of living a healthy life

1 NUTRITIOUS FOOD
Eat a balanced, healthy diet, rich in wholefoods and low in ultraprocessed foods.

2 STAY HYDRATED
Drink plenty of water to enable the body to perform at its best.

3 MANAGE STRESS
Being able to cope with everyday problems and situations is important.

4 PHYSICAL ACTIVITY
Get enough exercise, including cardio, strength and flexibility work.

5 LIMIT ALCOHOL
Drinking too much alcohol can negatively impact your overall health.

6 AVOID DRUGS
Including tobacco! Drugs have a negative effect on your health.

7 GOOD SOCIAL CONNECTIONS
Have healthy relationships in your life.

8 ENGAGE IN HOBBIES
Do things that you enjoy regularly.

9 LISTEN TO YOUR BODY
Know when something isn't right and seek help if needed.

10 HAVE ENOUGH SLEEP
Get consistent, good-quality sleep every day.

---

the normal parameters, and it can be a good idea to have a check-up every so often to see how your body is coping and to catch any problems early on.

Some signs of good health are mental rather than physical. If your brain is functioning optimally and there are no underlying conditions, you should be able to concentrate well, remember things with relative ease, and control your interactions and emotions. You should find that you're able to make decisions, let go of negativity and stay focused.

BONE AND MUSCLE HEALTH

Good health means having healthy bones – they are the structural system for the whole body. Bones protect our organs and store important minerals that we need for our health, as well as producing red and white blood cells in the bone marrow. It's important to nourish and protect our skeleton throughout our life, and to build healthy and strong bones. Stronger bones in later life reduce the risk of breakages and falls.

Looking after them comes down to a combination of lifestyle factors. Bone health is maintained through regular exercise and a healthy, balanced diet, rich in calcium and vital vitamins. It's also important that bones get enough vitamin D. Things like smoking or drinking too much alcohol have a negative impact on bone density and ▶

are risk factors for future problems. Keeping at a healthy weight also helps our skeleton, as being underweight or overweight can increase the risk of things like osteoporosis. It's difficult to tell how good our bones are without having a bone density scan, so it's important to maintain them through a healthy lifestyle – the first sign of a problem with bones is often only found after a breakage.

You also need strong muscles for good health. If you struggle with lifting everyday items, then this can indicate that you need to do some work on building up your muscular health. Poor muscle health can make it harder to do normal things like walking up the stairs, feeling weak or struggling with balance.

Healthy muscles should be both strong and flexible. This means that you are able to perform daily activities with no problems and you are less likely to fall. Muscles start to deteriorate as we age, so keeping an eye on muscle health throughout your life can ensure that you get older with fewer health problems.

HEART HEALTH

It's really important to look after your heart, ensuring that it's both strong and resilient. Leading an overall healthy lifestyle is the best way to protect your heart, but it's also a good idea to know the signs of a healthy heart so that you can spot if there are any issues you need to look into.

Ideally, for an adult, you would have a steady resting heart rate of between 60 and 100 beats per minute. A lower heart rate normally indicates a healthy heart, but if it drops too low, or goes too high, it should be checked out. Blood pressure should also fall within the normal parameters, as this helps to keep the heart functioning properly. High blood pressure, or hypertension, indicates that the heart is under too much strain. Similarly, high cholesterol can increase the risk of heart disease and heart attacks.

If your heart is working well, you should be able to engage in regular exercise – you may have to build up from where you are, but regular activity works the heart and improves your cardiovascular fitness

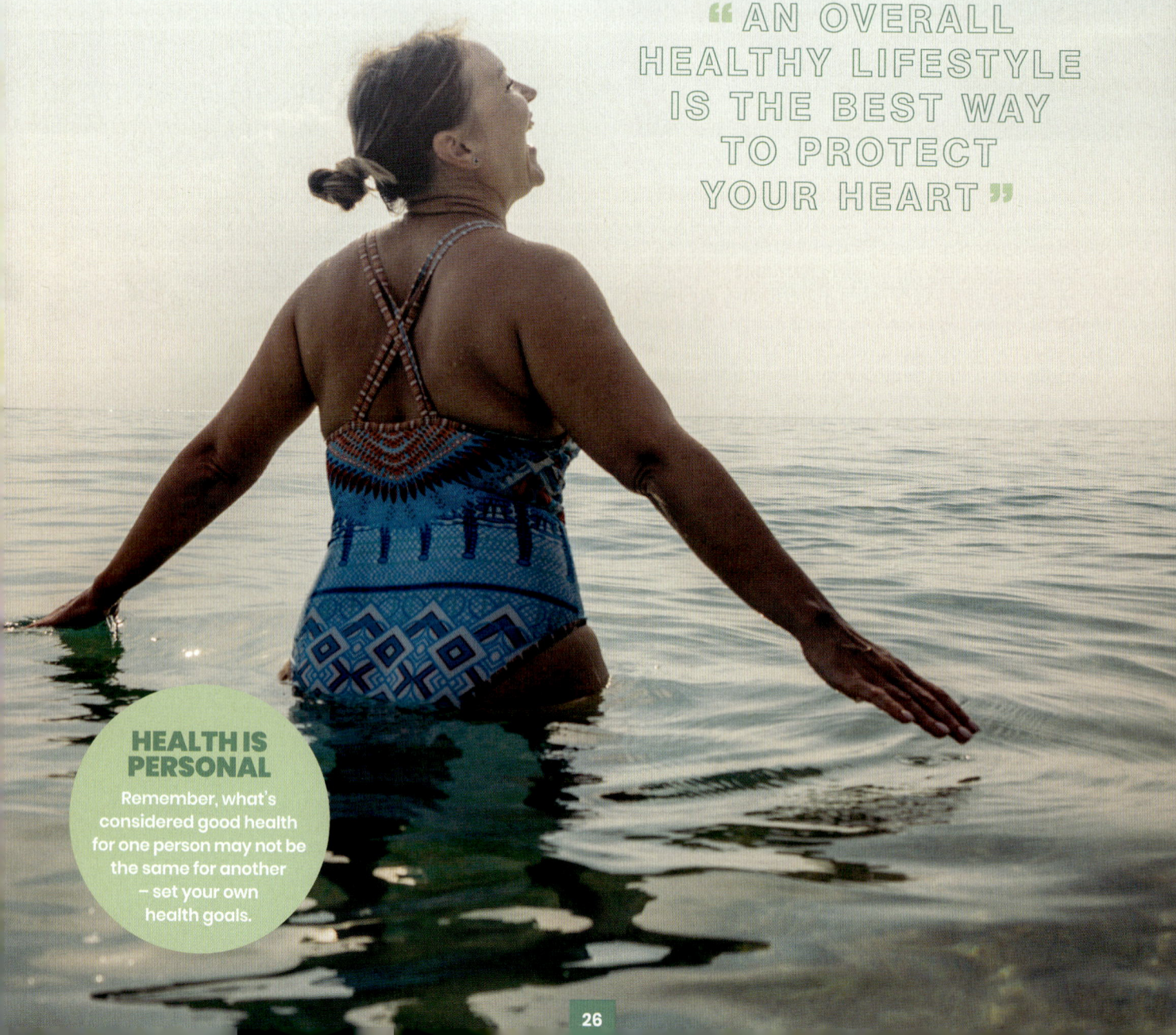

> "AN OVERALL HEALTHY LIFESTYLE IS THE BEST WAY TO PROTECT YOUR HEART"

HEALTH IS PERSONAL
Remember, what's considered good health for one person may not be the same for another – set your own health goals.

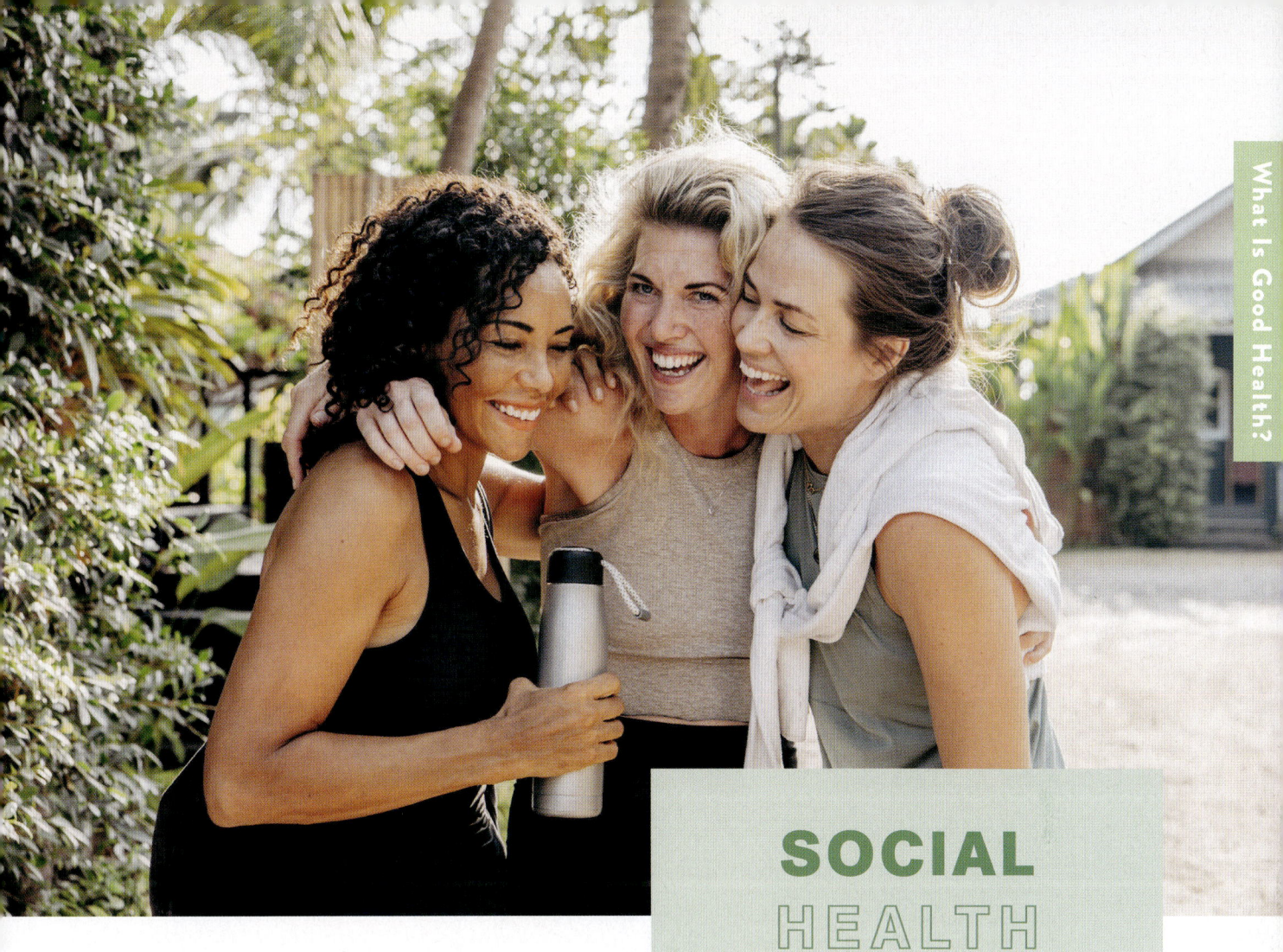

and strength. A strong heart also circulates the blood around the body; if your circulation isn't working as well as it should, you may notice that your fingers and toes lose colour and take on a blue or purple tinge.

IMMUNITY

Good health is linked to having a strong immune system. This enables your body to fight off infections and heal injuries faster. If you have a strong immune system then you may get ill less frequently, but when you do get ill you make a quicker recovery. A good immune system also means that you're less likely to find you suffer from some allergies.

Getting injured or having cuts and bruises is quite normal, but with a strong immune system you're likely to heal far more quickly and be back on your feet in no time. Your immune system is supported through a healthy lifestyle – water, sleep, nutrition, vitamins, minerals, gut health and low stress.

Chances are that reading through this list of good health indicators, you've mentally sorted them into 'yes' and 'no' piles. If you're seeking optimal health and wellbeing, then it's a good idea to focus on the areas where you're not exhibiting these positive signs – and where there are no underlying reasons why you can't make changes to improve.

SOCIAL HEALTH

Good health doesn't just relate to your mind and body; social wellness is important to your wellbeing

We know that having good social connections can help you to maintain your mental health, but it also helps with your physical health too – a strong social network can boost your immune system. There are signs of positive *social* health. These include having a trusted network of friends and family – the overall number doesn't matter so much, as long as you have people you can talk to. Maintaining these relationships well is also a good sign of social health, as is being able to put in place and respect boundaries, being able to communicate well, and engaging in social activities. Looking after social health doesn't mean you should be around others all the time – you need time to yourself as well. Finding the right balance for you is critical for your overall health.

HEALTH
CONDITIONS

Ten common health conditions that can impact women of all ages

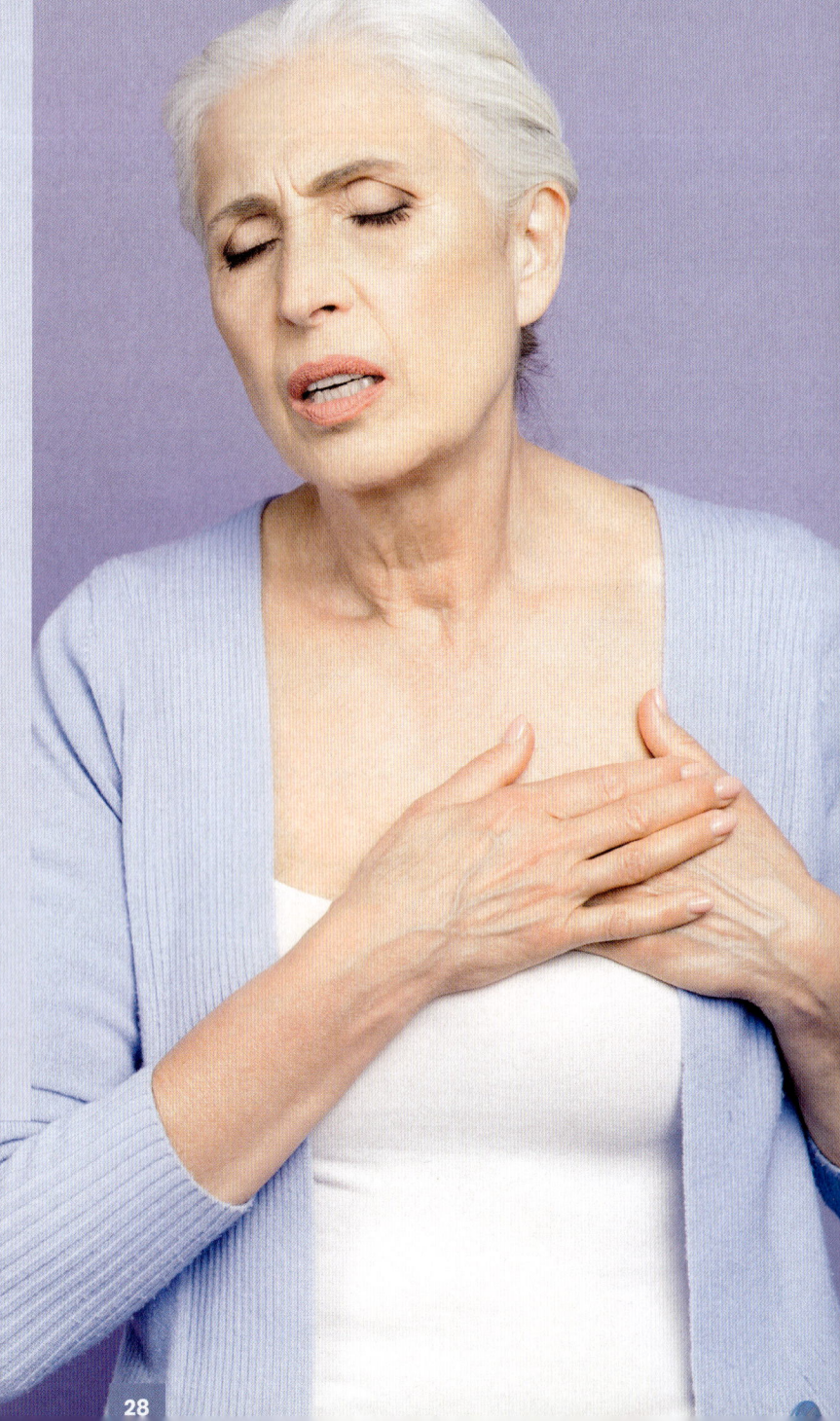

HEART DISEASE

Heart disease, or cardiovascular disease (CVD), is one of the biggest causes of death globally, and more than half a billion people around the world are affected.[1] The most common type is coronary heart disease (CHD). It tends to be thought of as an issue that mostly affects men, and while it's true that more men are diagnosed with heart disease than women, there is a gender gap in diagnosis and care, meaning that women might not receive treatment as quickly, leading to more serious outcomes.[2] Coronary heart disease can lead to a heart attack, a serious medical event. Knowing the signs of heart disease and a heart attack could save your life. Watch out for chest pain that doesn't go away, pain that spreads to one or both arms, shortness of breath, feeling dizzy or faint, feeling or being sick, sweating, sudden anxiety, and coughing and wheezing. If you're worried call the emergency services – the earlier treatment is received, the less damage that is done to the heart. Risk factors for heart disease include high blood pressure or cholesterol, diabetes, smoking, obesity, lack of exercise and a family history.

ACT FAST
If you're concerned about symptoms, don't leave it – early diagnosis can help with positive outcomes.

DIABETES

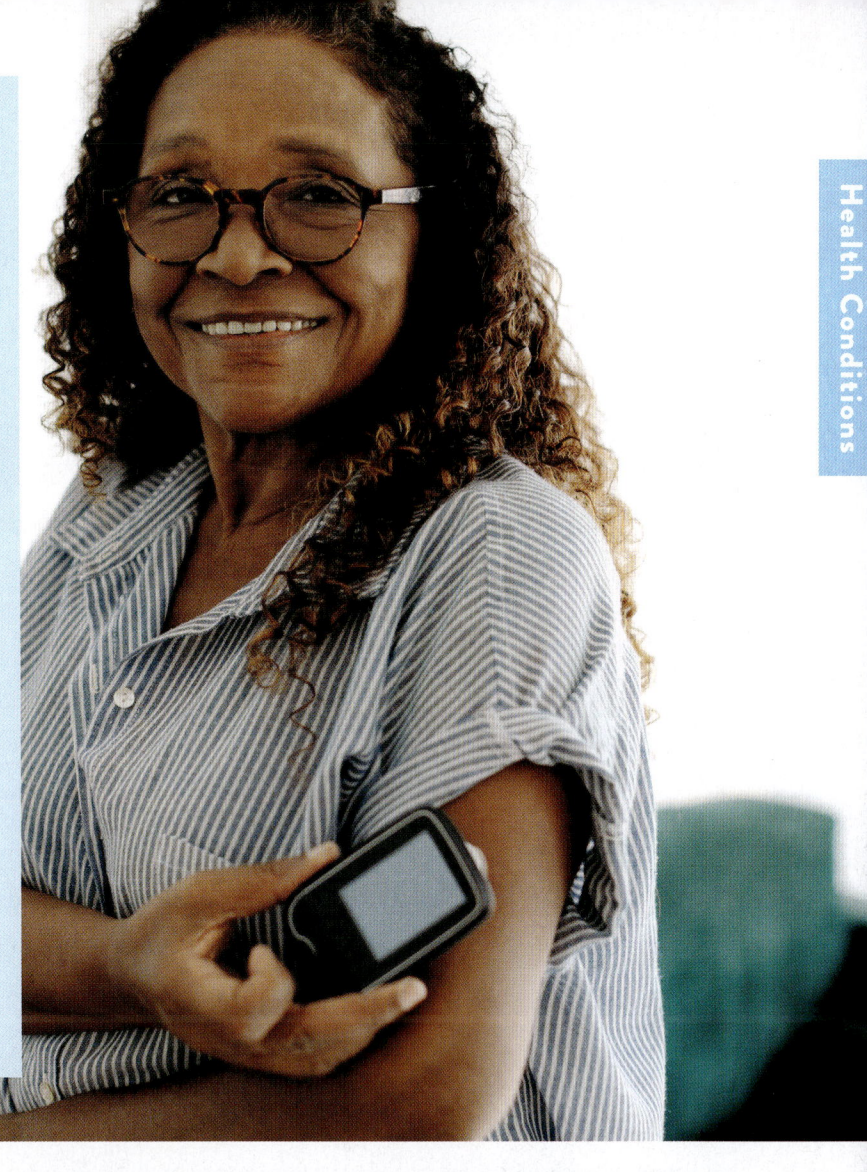

Diabetes is a condition in which a person's blood-sugar level is too high – and this can lead to serious complications. There are two types of diabetes. Type 1 diabetes is a lifelong condition, meaning that a person develops it typically in early childhood or during the pre-teen/early teenage years, though it can develop at any age. Type 1 diabetes means that the body's immune system destroys the cells that produce insulin. Type 2 diabetes is when the body doesn't produce enough insulin or the body's cells don't react to insulin as they should. Over 90% of adults who have diabetes will have type 2,[3] which can be triggered by lifestyle factors, unlike type 1 diabetes. The biggest risk factors for type 2 diabetes are being overweight or obese, a poor diet, being inactive, a family history of the disease or high blood pressure. Some ethnicities including Asian, Black African and African Caribbean are also at higher risk. Symptoms to watch out for include being very thirsty, urinating more than usual and especially at night, fatigue and blurred vision.

STROKE

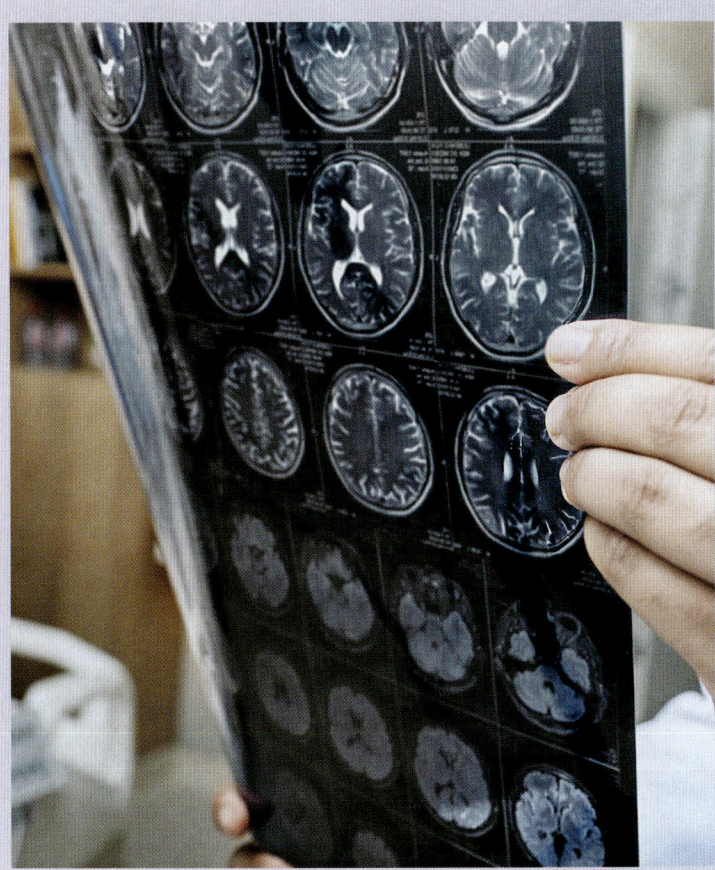

Stroke is another condition that is often thought of in terms of its impact in men. It's true that more men than women have strokes, but a stroke is still one of the four leading causes of death for women.[4] Women are also more likely to have strokes at a later age than men. For both sexes, risk factors include high blood pressure, high cholesterol, diabetes, smoking or inactivity. However, there are some risk factors that only impact women, including the use of the combined contraceptive pill in some women, pregnancy (though this is rare) and lupus. The risk of stroke in women begins to rise after menopause due to the lowering of hormone levels; women who have an early or medical menopause will also have an increased risk due to decreased oestrogen production. It's important to know the symptoms of a stroke: these include face weakness on one side of the face, arm weakness and slurred speech. ▸

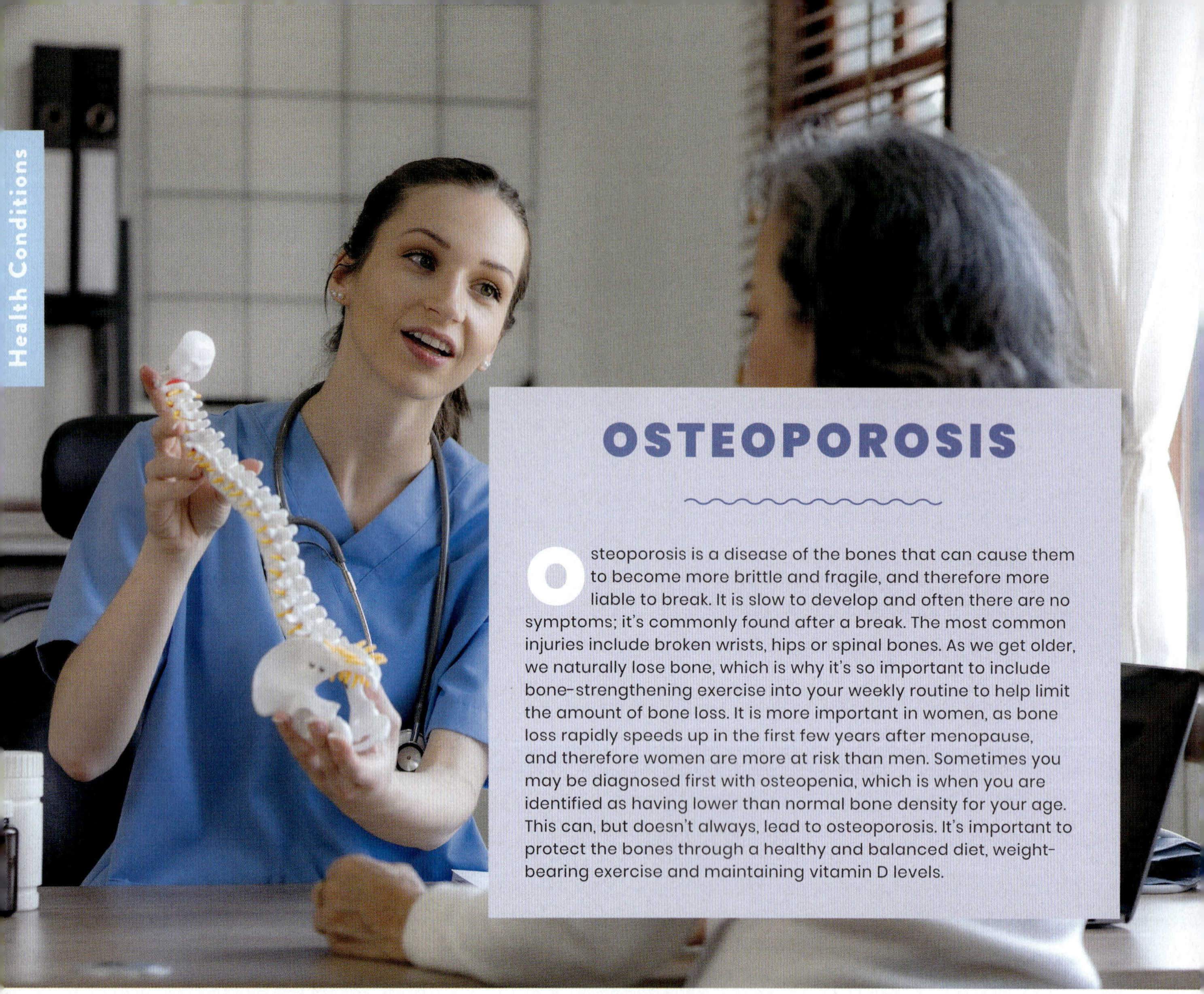

OSTEOPOROSIS

Osteoporosis is a disease of the bones that can cause them to become more brittle and fragile, and therefore more liable to break. It is slow to develop and often there are no symptoms; it's commonly found after a break. The most common injuries include broken wrists, hips or spinal bones. As we get older, we naturally lose bone, which is why it's so important to include bone-strengthening exercise into your weekly routine to help limit the amount of bone loss. It is more important in women, as bone loss rapidly speeds up in the first few years after menopause, and therefore women are more at risk than men. Sometimes you may be diagnosed first with osteopenia, which is when you are identified as having lower than normal bone density for your age. This can, but doesn't always, lead to osteoporosis. It's important to protect the bones through a healthy and balanced diet, weight-bearing exercise and maintaining vitamin D levels.

HYPERTENSION

Hypertension, or high blood pressure, is one of the biggest risks for heart disease and stroke, and yet it's one of the most preventable and treatable too. High blood pressure is more common in men for most of their lifetime, but after the age of 65 it's more common in women. It's really important to have regular blood pressure checks to catch any signs of a rise as early as possible – many pharmacies offer walk-in blood pressure checks, or you can get machines to test at home. High blood pressure rarely causes symptoms in the early stages and the only way you would know is by having a blood pressure check. In a very small number of cases, very high blood pressure can cause headaches, nosebleeds and blurred vision. However, if it's left untreated it can lead to kidney failure, heart failure, eyesight problems and vascular dementia. Rick factors include age, family history, smoking, drinking too much alcohol, eating too much salt, inactivity and being overweight.

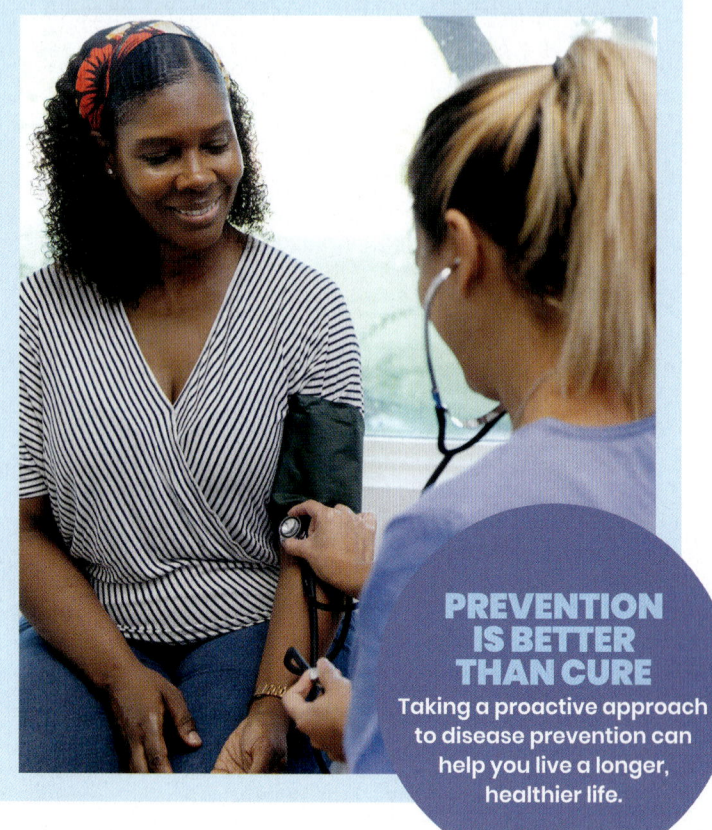

PREVENTION IS BETTER THAN CURE
Taking a proactive approach to disease prevention can help you live a longer, healthier life.

HEADACHES & MIGRAINES

It's quite common to experience headaches from time to time, which can be caused by anything from not being hydrated enough to being under a lot of stress. Migraines can feel like very bad headaches and are often on one side of the head. Migraines and headaches can be linked with hormonal changes in the body, which is why women may experience more pain before or during their period. Mostly, they can be treated with over-the-counter painkillers, and some women find that they need to use a cooling pad on their head or lie down in a darkened room. There are other medications and treatments for those who have very bad migraines regularly. Sometimes, lifestyle changes can help, particularly reducing caffeine intake or ensuring that you eat at regular intervals. Menopause can lead to a worsening of headaches and migraines, but many women find that post-menopause, they actually reduce in frequency.

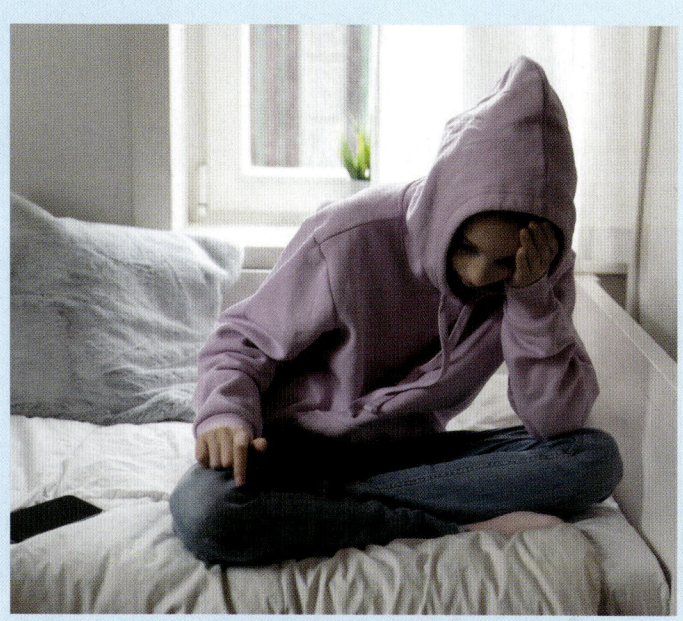

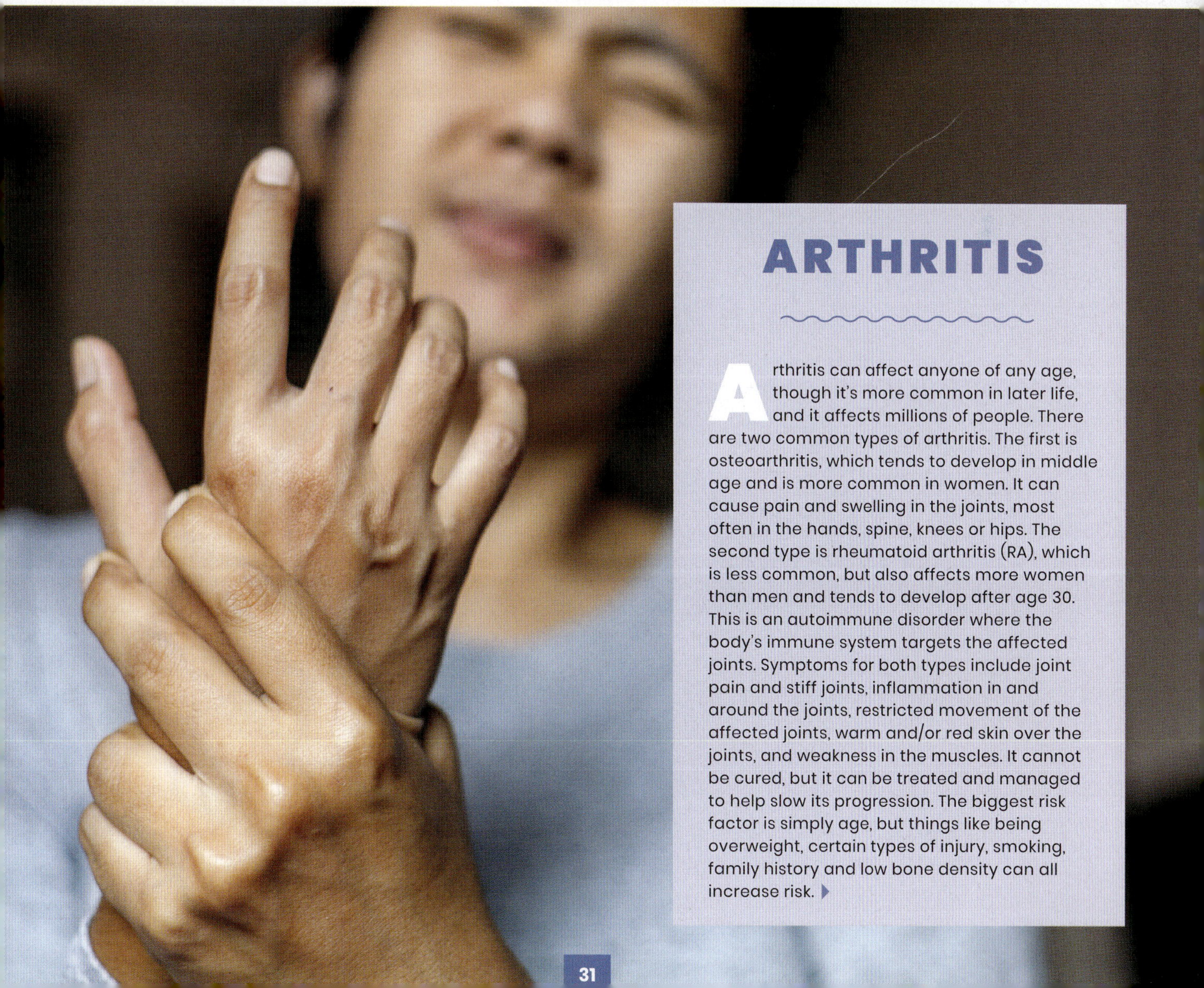

ARTHRITIS

Arthritis can affect anyone of any age, though it's more common in later life, and it affects millions of people. There are two common types of arthritis. The first is osteoarthritis, which tends to develop in middle age and is more common in women. It can cause pain and swelling in the joints, most often in the hands, spine, knees or hips. The second type is rheumatoid arthritis (RA), which is less common, but also affects more women than men and tends to develop after age 30. This is an autoimmune disorder where the body's immune system targets the affected joints. Symptoms for both types include joint pain and stiff joints, inflammation in and around the joints, restricted movement of the affected joints, warm and/or red skin over the joints, and weakness in the muscles. It cannot be cured, but it can be treated and managed to help slow its progression. The biggest risk factor is simply age, but things like being overweight, certain types of injury, smoking, family history and low bone density can all increase risk. ▸

RESPIRATORY CONDITIONS

There are a lot of different health conditions that can impact breathing function or the lungs. One of the most common is asthma, which is more common and more severe in women than men. It's thought that this could be linked to hormones, as many women experience worse symptoms around menstruation, but we don't yet know why.[5] Symptoms can also be worse during pregnancy and menopause, and asthma can be impacted by taking HRT. Common symptoms include wheezing, chest tightness, coughing, fast breathing or breathlessness, and a quickening heartbeat. It can begin at any age, usually in childhood, but it can also come on in adulthood.

Other respiratory conditions include chronic obstructive pulmonary disease (COPD), which affects the airways, and cystic fibrosis, which affects the lungs.

Untreated respiratory diseases and infections can lead to serious complications, so if you are struggling with breathing, chest pain, wheezing or coughing, you should always seek medical advice.

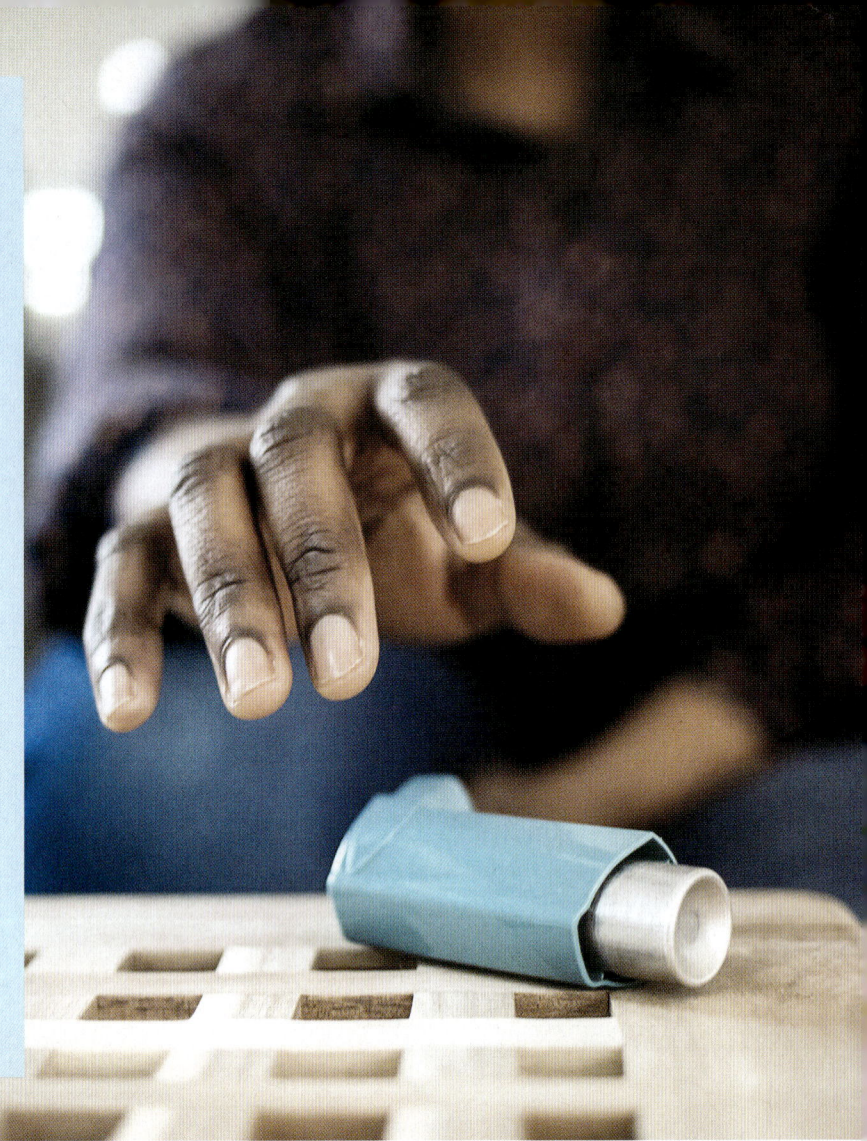

ORAL HEALTH CONDITIONS

We don't think much about the health of our mouth, but it's actually very important to look after it. Most oral health conditions are preventable and treatable, but when left can cause further health problems. Having oral health issues can affect your self-esteem and confidence, cause pain, and make it difficult to sleep. Poor oral health has even been linked to other health conditions, such as diabetes, stroke and heart disease. Tooth decay can occur through consuming too much sugar, which reacts with the bacteria in our mouths, which can then attack the teeth and cause small holes. This acid can also erode the surface of the teeth, leading to sensitivity and pain. The gums can become inflamed, sore and red, and start to bleed – all signs of gum disease. Good oral hygiene can help with these conditions, as can a healthy diet and a reduction in sugar intake.

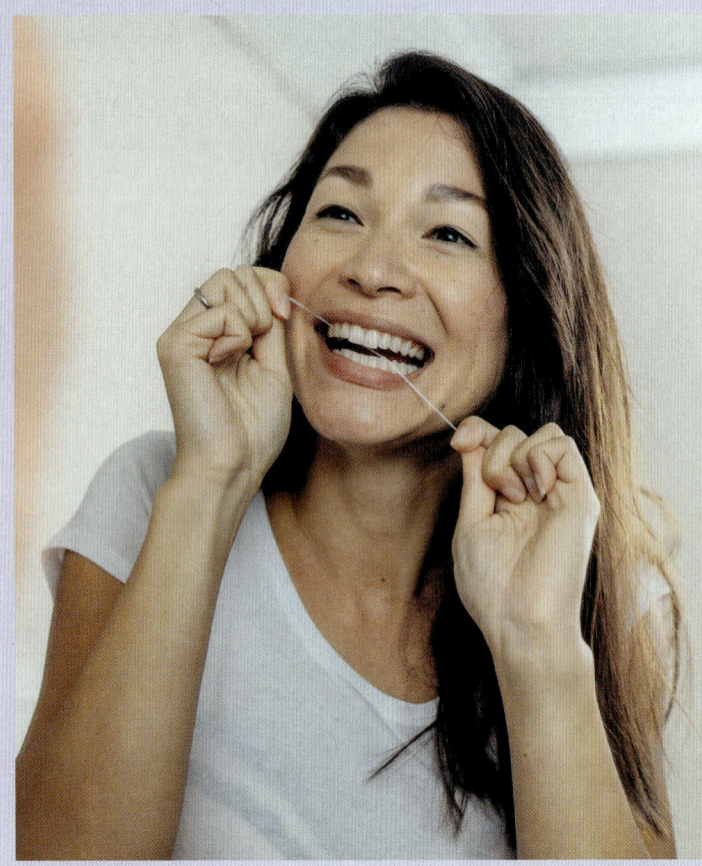

AUTOIMMUNE CONDITIONS

Women are more likely to have autoimmune diseases than men. One theory is that it's down to a molecule made by one of the X chromosomes that can trigger antibodies against a woman's tissues.[6] Autoimmune conditions are disorders where the immune system attacks a person's own body, causing a range of symptoms. Common autoimmune conditions include rheumatoid arthritis (RA – see the separate box on this), lupus, multiple sclerosis, inflammatory bowel disease (IBD), psoriasis (an inflamed skin condition), celiac disease, Hashimoto thyroiditis (which can cause an underactive thyroid) and scleroderma (a disease in the connective tissue between the skin and blood vessels). There are many more that we haven't mentioned – there are more than 80 different autoimmune disorders. There are different symptoms depending on the type of condition, but many of them can cause fatigue, joint pain, fevers and skin rashes or irritations. If you don't feel right, it's always worth speaking to a doctor to try to find an underlying cause.

HEALTH CONDITIONS ARE COMMON
40% of adults in the UK had at least one longstanding illness or condition in 2021.

FITNESS & EXERCISE

Engaging in regular physical activity can help you feel fitter and stronger throughout your entire life

Being physically active is an incredibly important part of looking after your health and wellness. According to the World Health Organization, people who are not active enough have a 20-30% increased risk of death compared to people who are sufficiently active. And yet, 31% of adults and 80% of adolescents do not reach the recommended levels of physical activity.

It starts in childhood; children who are active have better health, better cognitive outcomes, improved mental health and reduced body fat. Throughout adulthood, being active can ensure you stay physically and mentally healthy, reducing your risk of major health conditions. Being physically fit can make it easier to cope with the demands of pregnancy and childbirth, as well as helping to relieve and reduce the symptoms of perimenopause and menopause.

BENEFITS OF EXERCISE

There are huge benefits to engaging in regular exercise, consisting of cardiovascular workouts to look after the heart, and strength workouts to

MOTIVATION VS CONSISTENCY

You can't rely on feeling motivated all the time to get moving

One of the biggest reasons people don't do enough exercise is that they don't have the motivation. When we first start a new exercise routine, it's all shiny and exciting, so motivation is high. This is why the gyms are so busy in January when everyone wants to kickstart their 'new year, new me' routines. But, come March, the gyms are emptier again. Relying simply on being motivated is setting yourself up to fail – no one is motivated all the time. What matters more is being consistent: turning up and doing the work even when you don't feel like it. Decide how many times you want to work out each week – and then stick to it. Make it a non-negotiable like any other important appointment in your diary. It's better to do a shorter session than no session at all. If you don't think you can manage your planned 5km run, for example, just pop your trainers on and leave the house. Start with a brisk walk, maybe trying running for half a mile, and see how you feel. Some days that might be enough, but at least you've been consistent and moved; other days you might get to the 5km and wonder why it was so hard to get started at all.

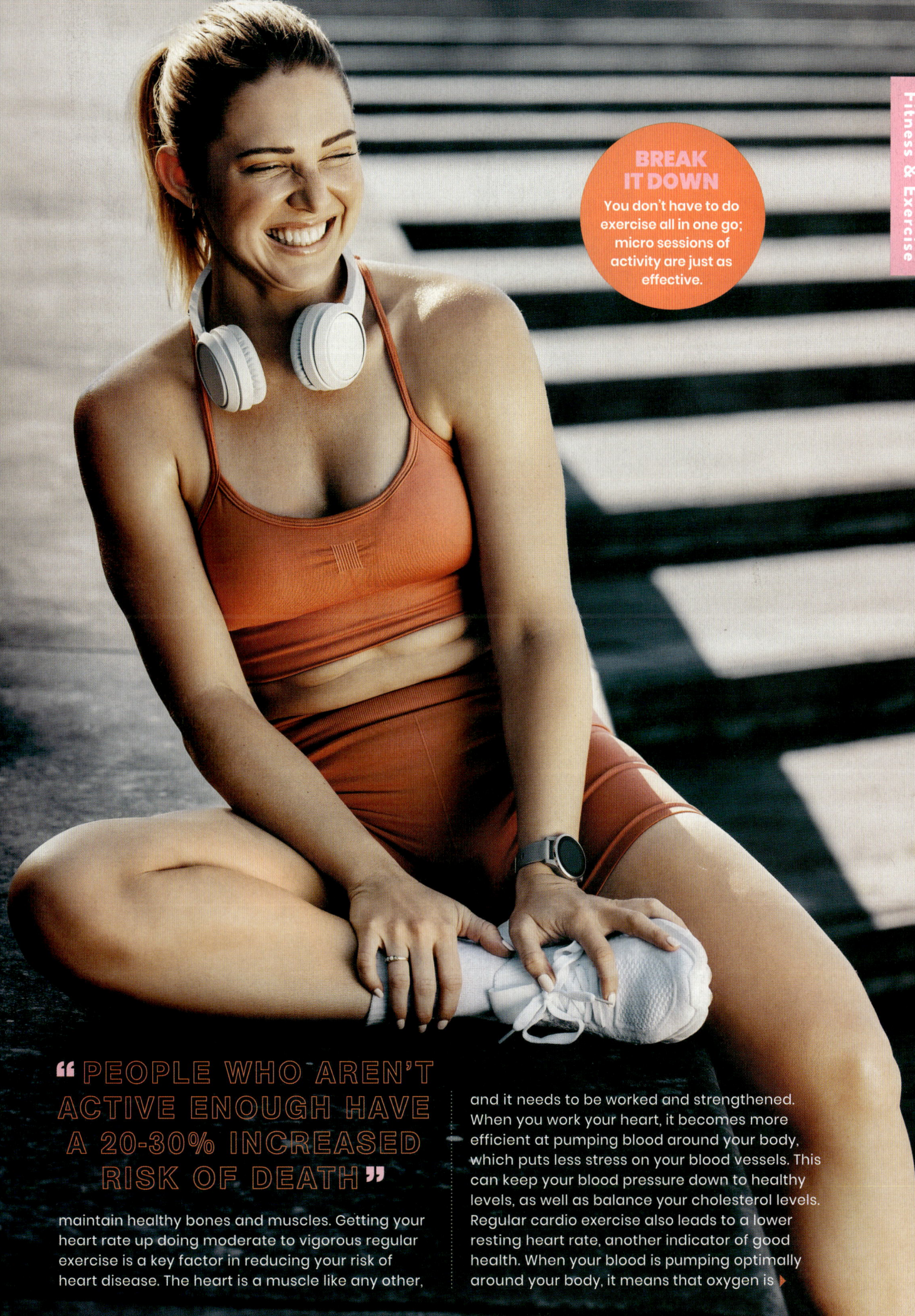

BREAK IT DOWN
You don't have to do exercise all in one go; micro sessions of activity are just as effective.

> **" PEOPLE WHO AREN'T ACTIVE ENOUGH HAVE A 20-30% INCREASED RISK OF DEATH "**

maintain healthy bones and muscles. Getting your heart rate up doing moderate to vigorous regular exercise is a key factor in reducing your risk of heart disease. The heart is a muscle like any other, and it needs to be worked and strengthened. When you work your heart, it becomes more efficient at pumping blood around your body, which puts less stress on your blood vessels. This can keep your blood pressure down to healthy levels, as well as balance your cholesterol levels. Regular cardio exercise also leads to a lower resting heart rate, another indicator of good health. When your blood is pumping optimally around your body, it means that oxygen is ▶

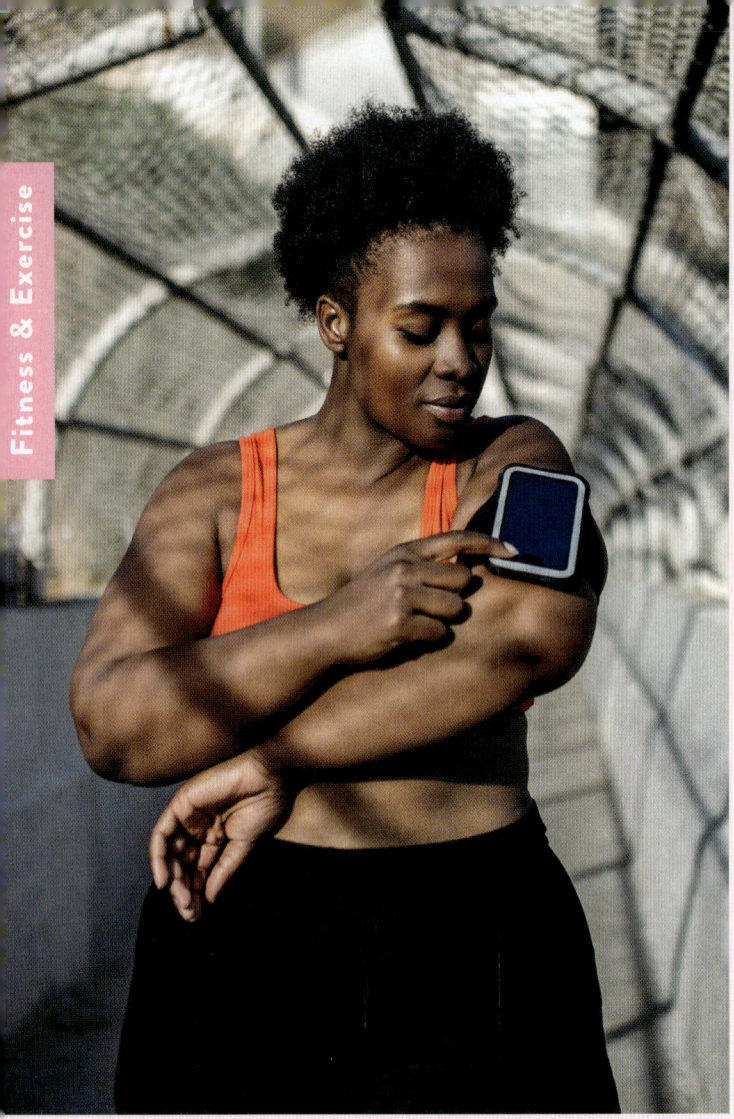

▶ reaching your tissues and organs, keeping them healthy, too.

It's not only your heart that benefits; your lungs do as well. As you exercise, you breathe more heavily and this can strengthen the muscles around the lungs, such as the diaphragm. This improves your lung function, meaning that you can take in more oxygen and deliver it to your muscles. Over time, your lungs will get stronger, so you can work at a harder intensity without getting breathless, giving you more stamina and enabling you to get fitter. Regular activity can also help with maintaining a healthy weight, which puts less pressure on your lungs and muscles, as well as reducing your risk of conditions like type 2 diabetes, heart disease and stroke.

Exercise can help you to sleep better by reducing stress hormones in the body, making you feel calmer and more in control. It's as good for our mental health as it is our physical, lifting mood and boosting self-esteem. It is so good for your mood that doctors often prescribe some form of movement as treatment for anxiety and depression, especially if combined with being outside in the fresh air.

Incorporating some strength work, whether that's bodyweight, weight-bearing or weightlifting, helps to protect your bone strength. Your bone density will drop as you get older, but the sooner you start looking after your bones, the less severe the impact. Strength work also helps to create strong, lean muscle. This makes your metabolism more efficient, which can help to maintain weight, as well as improve your overall body composition. As you go through menopause, strength training helps to offset the natural decline in muscle mass. Strength training, in conjunction with mobility work, can also improve balance, which can prevent falls and injuries in later life.

CARDIO EXERCISE

Cardiovascular exercise, or just 'cardio', is any type of exercise that gets your heart pumping. You might think doing cardio means slogging through a group exercise class you don't like, or running when you'd rather do anything but! Both of those are great cardio options, of course, but the key is to make sure you do something that's right for you. That means something you like, something that fits into your life, something that fits your budget and something you'll stick to.

> **"THE KEY IS TO DO SOMETHING THAT'S RIGHT FOR YOU, THAT FITS INTO YOUR LIFE"**

If you can, some of your cardio should be done outside. The benefits of being outside in nature are well known, helping to reduce blood pressure, improve mental health and lower stress levels. Going for a walk or run in your local area, doing a bootcamp in the park, or even going for a chilly swim in the sea are all going to give you a lot of health benefits.

You may not always be able to, or want to, exercise outside, but there are a lot of inside options too. You could go to the gym, join in with an aerobics or indoor cycling class, or even follow an at-home workout on your television. If you're new to exercise, you might feel a little self-conscious. Some women like to get used to different types of exercise at home first before taking it into a more public environment. Your body doesn't know the difference, though – it just needs to be moved in a way that suits you.

Intensity matters when it comes to cardio. Cardio should fall into either the moderate or vigorous activity categories. Moderate exercise is just enough to make your breathing go faster, but you can still hold a conversation. This includes things like brisk walking, cycling or lower-intensity gym classes. If something is vigorous, you will be breathing harder and faster, making it difficult to talk. This includes things like running, high-intensity interval training (HIIT), circuits and team sports. As well as this more intense activity, you should be trying to increase the amount of everyday 'normal' activity that you do. This is called NEAT – non-exercise activity thermogenesis – which is the energy you expend just living your life. This includes sitting, standing, walking, doing household jobs, playing with your children, gardening and so on. It's still physical activity, but it's not prescribed exercise. You can improve your fitness a great deal by making sure you do more NEAT activities every day.

Just because cardio is important and needs a level of intensity, it doesn't mean it has to be high impact. Things like running and jumping put a lot of pressure on the joints and muscles, which doesn't suit everyone. Lower-impact activity like walking and swimming can get your heart rate up adequately, while looking after your body.

BUILDING YOUR STRENGTH

One of the best things you can do for your body, alongside your cardio workouts, is make sure you're including some strength work at least a couple of times a week. This is important throughout your life to help look after your muscles and bones, but it becomes even more important as you age. Throughout perimenopause and menopause, when your bone density and muscle mass start to decline, regular strength training can slow down the progression of this loss, while helping to keep your body strong and lean. Beyond menopause and into later life, it can help you to stay independent and less likely to suffer from falls or health problems.

PHYSICAL ACTIVITY GUIDELINES

How much exercise should you be doing each week?

As adults, there are guidelines set out by health authorities that outline the minimum recommended amount of physical activity we should be doing every week. These are broadly the same around the world and apply to all adults aged 19 to 64 years old. If you have a disability or health condition, you may need to make some adaptations, but it's still important to be active. You can also exercise throughout pregnancy, if you're not advised otherwise, and in the post-partum period, following your doctor's advice.

• Do at least 150 minutes of moderate intensity activity every week, or 75 minutes of vigorous intensity activity every week.

• Do strength exercises covering all the major muscle groups at least two days a week.

• Break up sedentary periods of sitting or lying down by ensuring you stand up and move around.

• Include strength and flexibility exercises every week.

For children aged 5 to 18 years old, the aim is to do at least 60 minutes of moderate or vigorous-intensity activity a day, which should include a variety of types of movement spread out over the day, as well as reducing the time spent sitting or lying down. Older adults – those over 65 – should still aim to meet the adult guidelines, but if you're not able to, then it's important to do at least some light activity every day.

STAND UP
If you have to sit a lot at work, try to make sure you stand up regularly and move around.

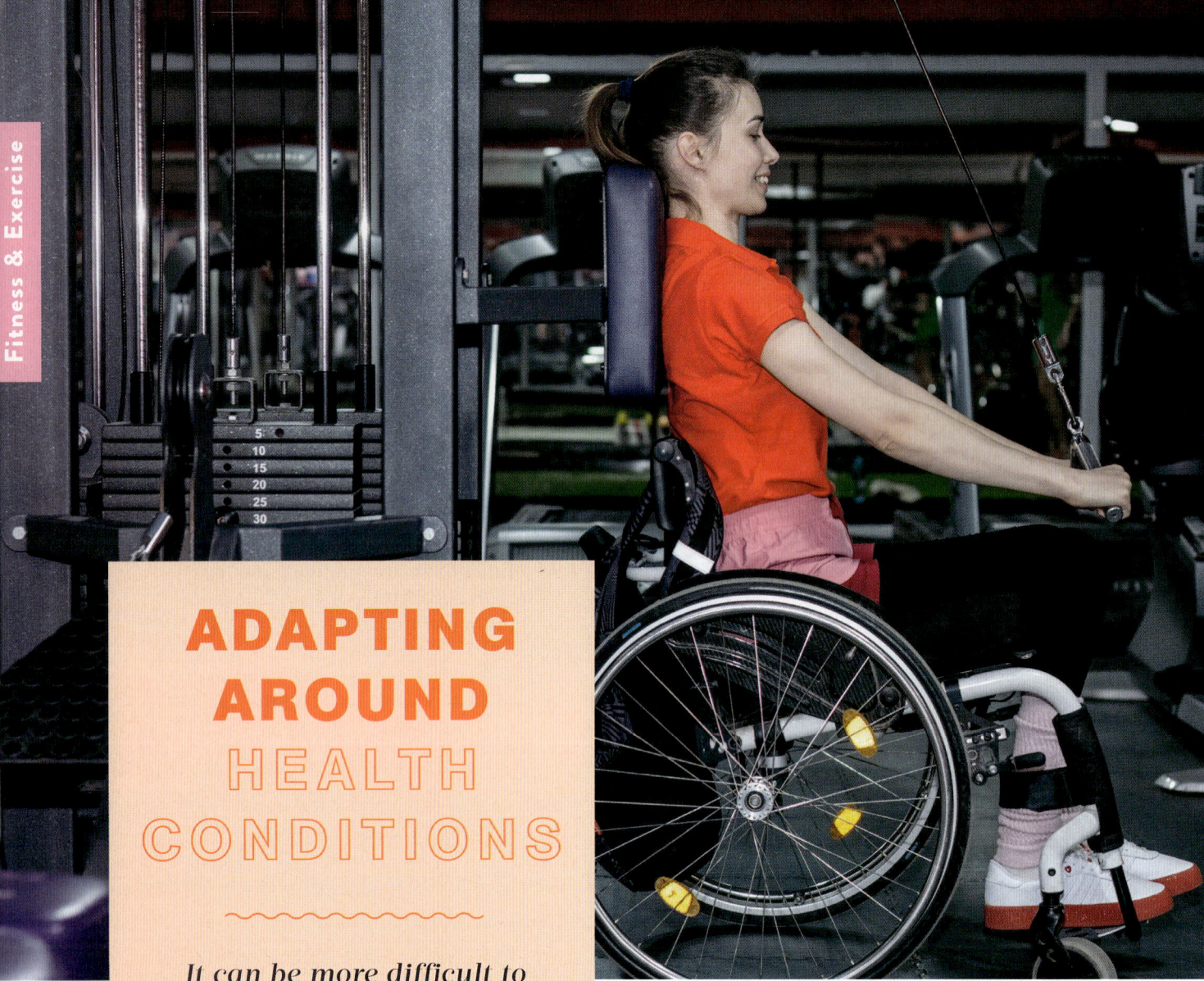

ADAPTING AROUND HEALTH CONDITIONS

It can be more difficult to exercise if you have underlying health conditions or a disability

There can be challenges to being physically active, which can mean it's harder to take part in certain forms of exercise. There are a lot of adaptations and types of exercise that might still suit, so you should be able to find something that works for you. You may need to get advice from your doctor before you engage in new activity, but it's important to try to be as physically active as you are able to be, to ensure you stay fit and healthy. Have a look at what's available in your local area – there are often exercise classes aimed at those living with a disability or long-term health condition. This can be everything from badminton to chair yoga, or swimming to weight training. There are also personal trainers who specialise in aiding those with health conditions, as well as adapted areas within gyms that offer more inclusive workout options.

▶ Strength training doesn't have to be just picking up heavy weights. You can use your own body weight and resistance machines, as well as free weights. Bodyweight workouts are great for beginners, but they are also good for women of all levels of experience. They don't need any equipment, so it's very accessible to everyone and you can pretty much do it anywhere with minimal space requirements. There are plenty of freely available workouts online, so it doesn't have to cost anything either. Bodyweight exercises include things like squats, lunges, press-ups, planks and sit-ups, among others. There are always ways to adapt the exercises to meet your current strength level. So, for example, you might do press-ups on your knees or on an incline, and progress towards full press-ups. You can work your whole body and multiple muscle groups at a time, using nothing more than your own body.

You may also want to start incorporating free weights, such as dumbbells, a barbell with plates, or a kettlebell. You can do all the same bodyweight exercises, just with some extra resistance, as well as different forms of exercise such as chest presses, deadlifts and bicep curls. Again, you can do this at home with instructional videos, but you

> "ONE THING THAT'S OFTEN NEGLECTED IS FLEXIBILITY AND STRENGTH WORK"

may want to consider doing a group class or a one-on-one PT session if you're new to weights to make sure your form is good to prevent injury. Using a gym also means you don't have to invest in weights of your own, and you can progress up through the weights as you get stronger. If you're a beginner, don't overlook simple resistance bands, which are cheap and portable, and can be highly effective. At the gym you can also access resistance machines. They often have instructions on them to help you get started. You can adjust the weight to suit your level and progress as time goes on.

FLEXIBILITY AND MOBILITY

One thing that's often neglected is flexibility and strength work, but it's so important. As we get older, our flexibility and mobility can decline, which can mean we find it harder to do normal, everyday activities and we're more at risk of falls. This is also something that can be impacted during menopause, as oestrogen helps to look after our connective tissues, ligaments and tendons. After menopause, these tissues might not regenerate as quickly as they did before, which can lead to stiffness and pain. But we can retain our mobility; like all exercise, the sooner you start, the greater the impact.

If you do a hard cardio or strength session, don't neglect the cooldown stretches – consider them an important part of the workout. We need to stretch the muscles we've used to help keep them flexible and aid in recovery.

Additionally, we should all be doing specific sessions every week dedicated to stretching and mobility. This could be through something like yoga, which helps with strength, flexibility and bone health. It also helps with your mental health and stress levels. You can follow videos to do this at home or join a group class for further instruction. Pilates is another option, helping to strengthen your whole body, but in particular your core strength. Pilates focuses on engaging your pelvic floor, keeping those muscles strong, which have huge benefits in pregnancy and recovering from childbirth, as well as helping with bladder control.

Being physically active and healthy means having a good balance of movement. Your weekly routine should, ideally, have elements of cardio workouts, strength training and flexibility work. And it should also have adequate periods of rest and recovery, which is just as important to prevent injury, overtraining and fatigue.

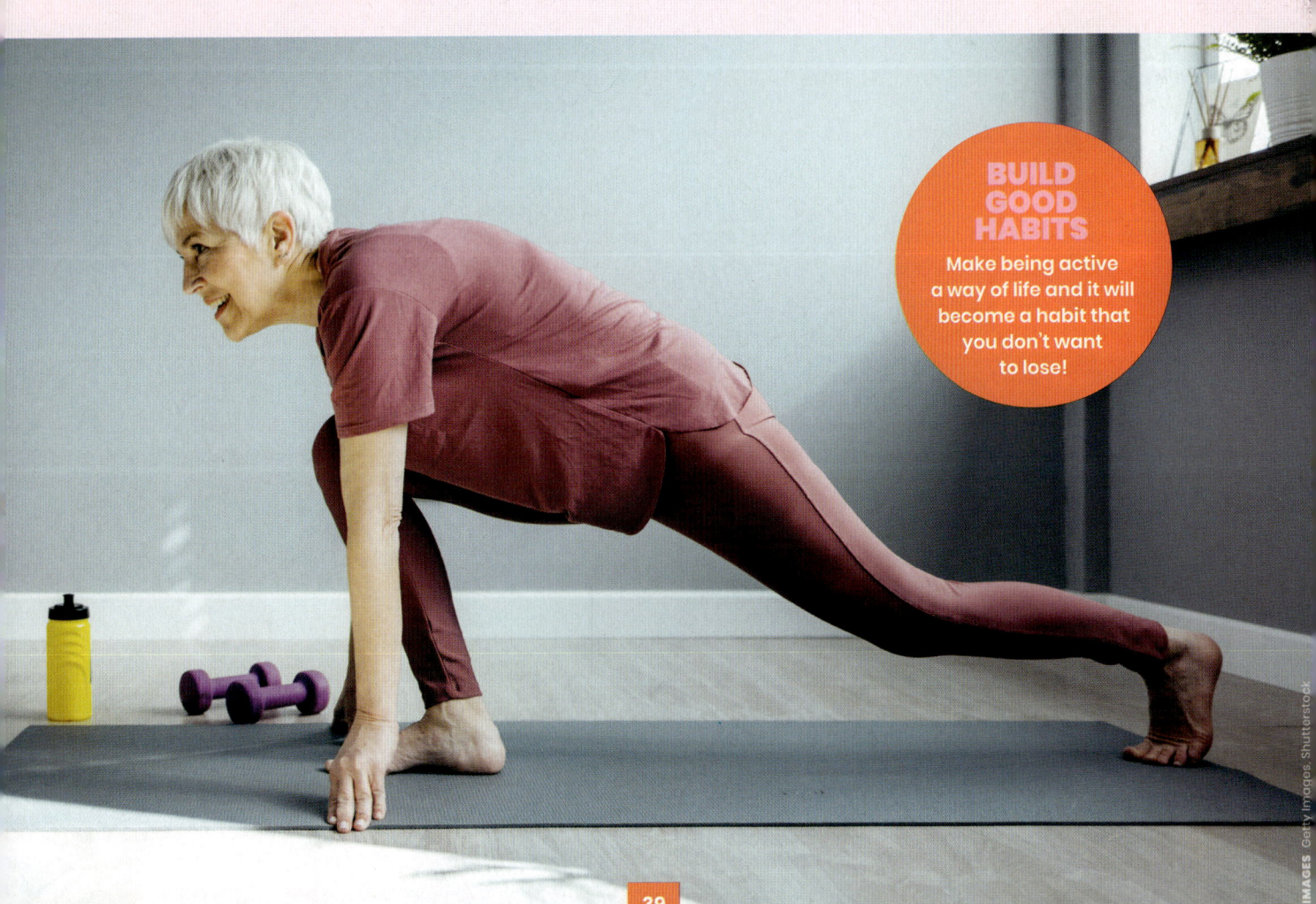

BUILD GOOD HABITS
Make being active a way of life and it will become a habit that you don't want to lose!

Diet & Nutrition

FOCUS ON FIBRE
We need at least 30g of fibre per day for optimal health, but in the UK and USA, the average intake is only 16–20g.

DIET & NUTRITION

A healthy, balanced diet is important to your overall health and wellbeing

Your diet can have a huge impact on the way you feel and is a significant contributor to being in good health. Unfortunately, it's easy to slip into bad habits with food and drink. We're busier than ever before, juggling long hours at work with children, family, partners, household admin, and trying to fit in exercise and a social life. When it comes to food, quick and convenient is often what we need.

The cost of healthy food can sometimes seem prohibitive, and then there is knowing what we should and shouldn't be eating. Nowadays there's so much information available around diet and nutrition, with thousands of experts at our fingertips, each telling us what we need to eat for our health – and they all contradict each other! Should you eat low-carb or low fat? Maybe keto is best for you – or a carnivore diet? When there is so much information, it's hard to filter through and make sense of it.

Sometimes you need to step back and trust your instincts. The more you get to know and understand your body, the easier it will be to figure out what works best for you. Most of us don't need another diet where food groups are restricted or encouraged, but rather a return to simple healthy eating.

BACK TO BASICS

There are some basics of nutrition that contribute to a healthy, balanced diet, which is key to our health. That balance comes from making sure we're eating enough of all three of the major macronutrients. You've probably heard of 'macros' when it comes to certain diet types, but all that means is the ratio you have between carbohydrates, fats and protein. We need all of these to help our body function properly.

> **"MOST OF US NEED A RETURN TO SIMPLE HEALTHY EATING"**

Carbohydrates give us energy, so these are important to enable us to do daily activities and exercise. The main source of carbohydrates are starchy foods such as cereals, bread, pasta, rice and potatoes. Despite the many popular low-carb diets, these foods play a key role in a healthy diet. Choose wholegrain varieties where possible, which break down more slowly, helping to release the energy in a controlled way. Carbohydrates are also a good source of fibre, of which many of us don't eat enough. Eating plenty of fibre is linked to a lower risk of some health conditions and may even reduce symptoms of depression, anxiety and stress. Fibre can make you feel fuller for longer, reducing cravings and helping to maintain a healthy weight. Starchy foods also contain important calcium, iron and B-vitamins.

Protein is important when it comes to building and maintaining your muscle mass, as well as helping you to feel fuller for longer. Most adults need about 0.75-1g of protein per ▶

kilo of body weight, but those who eat a typical Western diet are unlikely to be eating less than this anyway. You may need more protein if you're training regularly, especially if you lift a lot of heavy weights. What matters most is getting it from healthy, lean sources. That means opting for foods like lean meat and fish, eggs, soybeans, nuts and seeds, tofu and legumes, rather than highly processed meat products like sausages, burgers or sandwich meats. Ideally you want to eat a variety of different types of protein over the course of a week.

Finally, you also need to include fat in your diet. Fat has been demonised in the past, but we can't function without it! We need healthy fats to help with brain function and heart health, reducing the risk of cardiovascular disease. The type of fat we need is unsaturated, healthy fats, such as olive oil, avocados, nuts and fish, while limiting saturated fats. Fat also helps you to feel fuller for longer.

One of the best diets to follow, from a nutritional point of view, is the Mediterranean diet. It's not a restrictive diet and is a way of eating that ensures a balance of macros, along with vitamins and minerals. It is high in fruits, vegetables, wholegrains, legumes and pulses, nuts and seeds, plus healthy fats. It limits ultraprocessed foods, added sugar and refined grains. This mirrors the nutritional guidance given by most global health authorities for optimal health, including the Eatwell Guide in the UK and MyPlate in the USA.

If you have intolerances or allergies, it can be harder to eat a balanced diet, especially if it means eliminating a whole food group. You may wish to speak to a nutritionist or dietician to help plan a diet that works for you, ensuring you get a good variety of nutrients.

> **" MOST ADULTS DON'T CURRENTLY GET THEIR 'FIVE A DAY' "**

KEY MICRONUTRIENTS

Once you've covered the main macronutrients, you then need to make sure you're eating a variety of foods that will give you all the key vitamins and minerals your body needs. Each micronutrient helps your body function optimally, but by eating a lot of different fruits and vegetables, plus other plant foods – sometimes described as 'eating the rainbow' – you should already be eating most of these naturally.

However, many adults don't currently get their 'five a day' or a wide enough variety of plant foods. Whether you're a meat-eater, vegetarian or vegan, try to aim for 25 to 30 different plant foods in your menu each week.

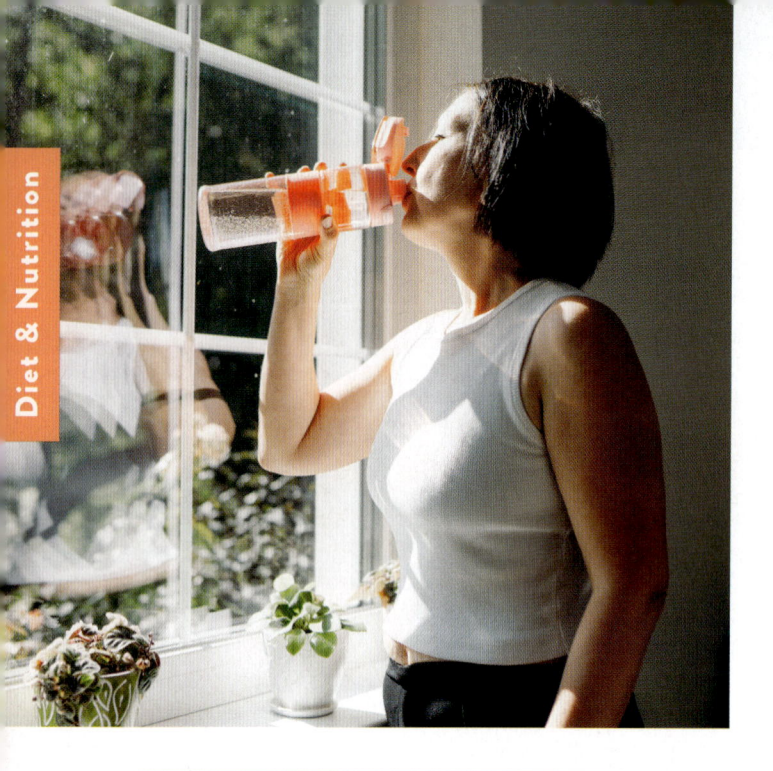

STAY HYDRATED

Alongside a healthy diet, it's also important to drink enough fluids

Do you drink enough water? Many of us don't, and yet it's really important for optimal health. Being well hydrated helps with digestion and in maintaining gut health, which can reduce the chance of constipation or developing urinary tract infections. Plenty of water also helps our skin to be healthy and glowing, as well as flexible. It contributes to good eye health, brain health and circulation. Water is best, rather than other fluids, but you can boost your fluid intake by eating water-rich foods like watermelon or cucumber, or drinking non-caffeinated herbal teas or low-sugar squash. Most people need about eight cups of water a day, which is about two litres, though if you're very active you may need more. This should be enough to keep your urine a pale yellow colour – a darker colour indicates you need to hydrate more. If you don't get enough water, you might want to try a tracker or a bottle that has markings on so you can visually see how much you need to drink.

Diet & Nutrition

One nutrient you do want to include is omega-3 fatty acid, which is good for your heart, brain and metabolic health. It can also help with lowering inflammation levels and looking after your joints. This can be found in oily fish, such as salmon or mackerel, as well as flaxseeds, walnuts and eggs. It's also important for women, particularly if you're of reproductive age and having regular periods, to have enough iron. Iron is critical to haemoglobin, which is found in red blood cells, and helps to transport oxygen around the body. Iron also helps with immune function, energy levels, and healthy skin and hair. Iron deficiency (anaemia) can cause heart palpitations, pale skin, headaches, shortness of breath and a lack of energy. Iron is found in animal products like red meat, poultry and seafood. Otherwise, you can get iron in legumes, dark leafy green vegetables, nuts and seeds, dried fruit, and foods fortified with iron. If you don't eat enough iron, you may need to consider a supplement.

If you're at the age when you're beginning perimenopause and struggling with some ▶

DIET IN PERIMENOPAUSE

As you get older, you may need to adapt your diet to suit your changing body

As you get older and reach perimenopause and menopause, you might need to make changes to your diet to help maintain your weight and to get the right nutrients to support your body through the transition. A healthy diet can also help to relieve symptoms. You may find that you need slightly fewer calories than pre-menopause as your metabolism slows down. You may also need to increase your protein intake a little, especially if you are strength training, to help retain muscle mass, as well as eat plenty of calcium and vitamin D for bone strength. The way your body responds to food in perimenopause can start to change. Research undertaken by ZOE (zoe.com) shows that women tend to experience less severe blood sugar spikes after eating compared to men pre-menopause. As we get older, our blood sugar levels after a meal start to increase more, which can lead to energy spikes and dips. Focusing on real, whole foods and a balanced overall diet is the best way to ensure good health through menopause and beyond.

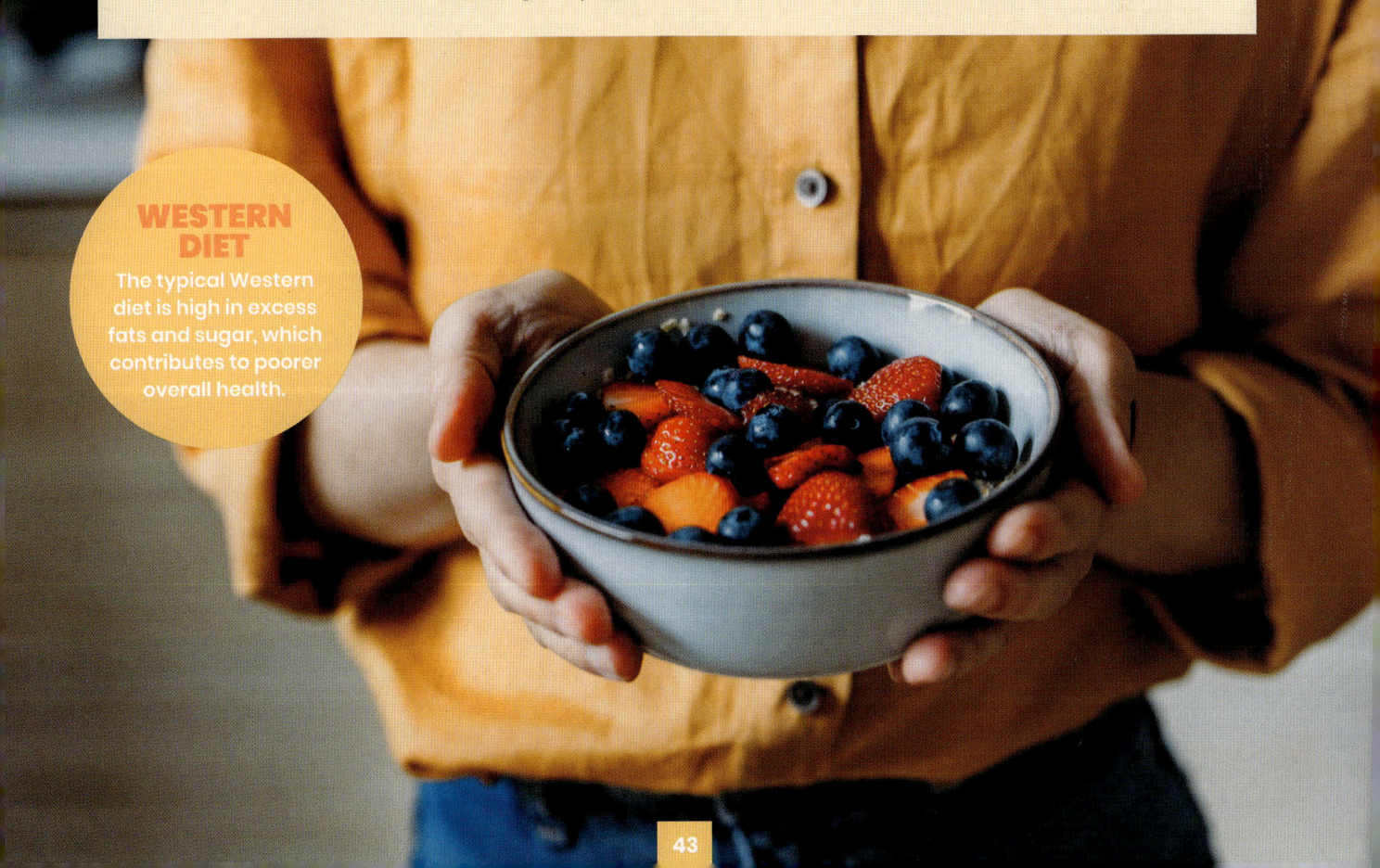

WESTERN DIET
The typical Western diet is high in excess fats and sugar, which contributes to poorer overall health.

CALCIUM FOR BONE STRENGTH

Make sure you get enough of this key mineral throughout your life

Calcium is important from childhood through to later life, especially when it comes to looking after our bones and teeth. This is even more so as we age, as we naturally start to lose calcium from our bones. Calcium-rich foods include milk, cheese, yogurt or milk-based puddings. If you're plant-based or vegan, you can get calcium-enriched dairy alternatives. There's also calcium in bread made with fortified flour, fish where you eat the bones (like sardines), and green leafy vegetables such as curly kale. Alongside calcium, we also need vitamin D, which helps with the absorption of the calcium. Some foods have small levels of vitamin D such as oily fish, red meat, liver, egg yolks and fortified foods. Most of our vitamin D comes from exposing our skin to sunlight. However, in countries where we don't get enough sunlight (such as in the UK between September and April), supplementation is recommended. All adults should take at least 10 micrograms a day, but it's still important to get outside and expose your skin to daylight for around ten minutes a day when you can – being careful not to burn!

symptoms, then you can include foods that are rich in phytoestrogens. These occur in plants and can give you 'oestrogen-like' effects, which may relieve some post-menopause symptoms. Examples of phytoestrogens are soy and linseed, which you can find in things like linseed bread, edamame beans, soy-enriched milk or yogurts, and soy-based foods like tofu, tempeh and miso.

Don't neglect your gut health, either. Poor gut diversity can be linked to all kinds of health conditions and inflammation in the body. Remember that your gut will love lots of fruits and vegetables, wholefoods and plant foods. You can also give your microbiome a boost by eating fermented and probiotic foods such as kimchi, kefir, miso, sauerkraut and Greek yogurt.

LESS-HEALTHY FOODS

At the same time as ensuring that you're eating enough healthy foods, it's also a good idea to limit the consumption of less-healthy foods. This doesn't mean cutting out all the foods you love; there is a place for everything in a balanced diet. The problem is when we eat these less-healthy foods all the time, which can directly impact on your health.

Try to avoid added sugar in products where you can. This can be harder than it sounds, as sugar hides under many different names, such as high-fructose corn syrup, corn sugar, sucrose, dextrose, glucose and maltose. It can also be present in products that you wouldn't expect to find it in, such as processed bread and bread products, soups,

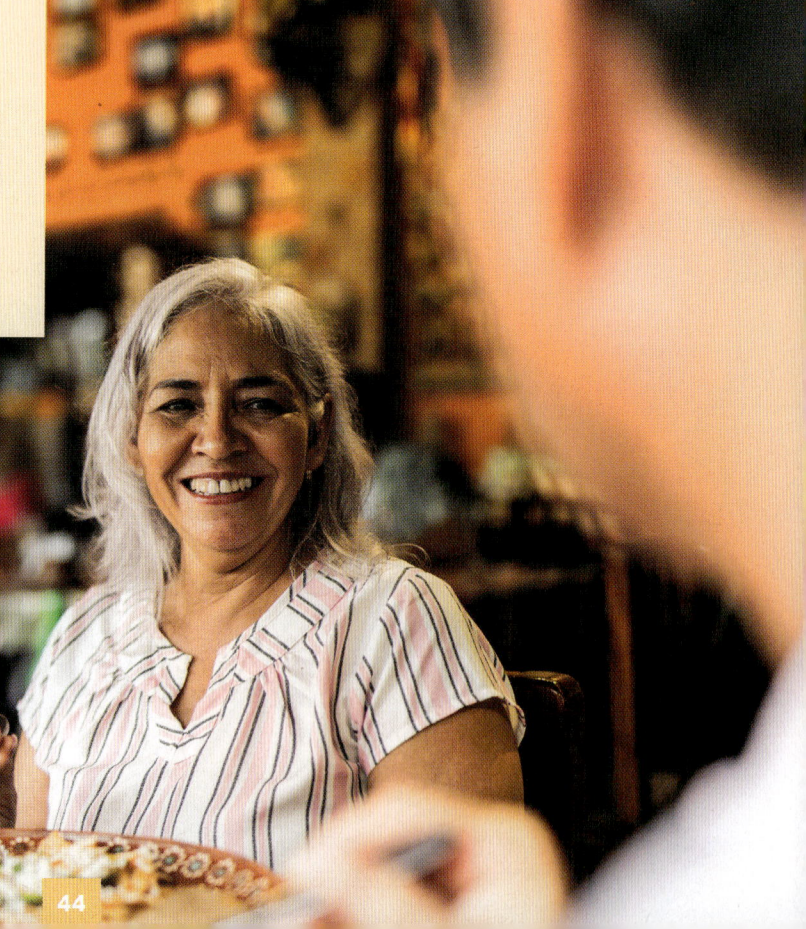

FOOD DIARY

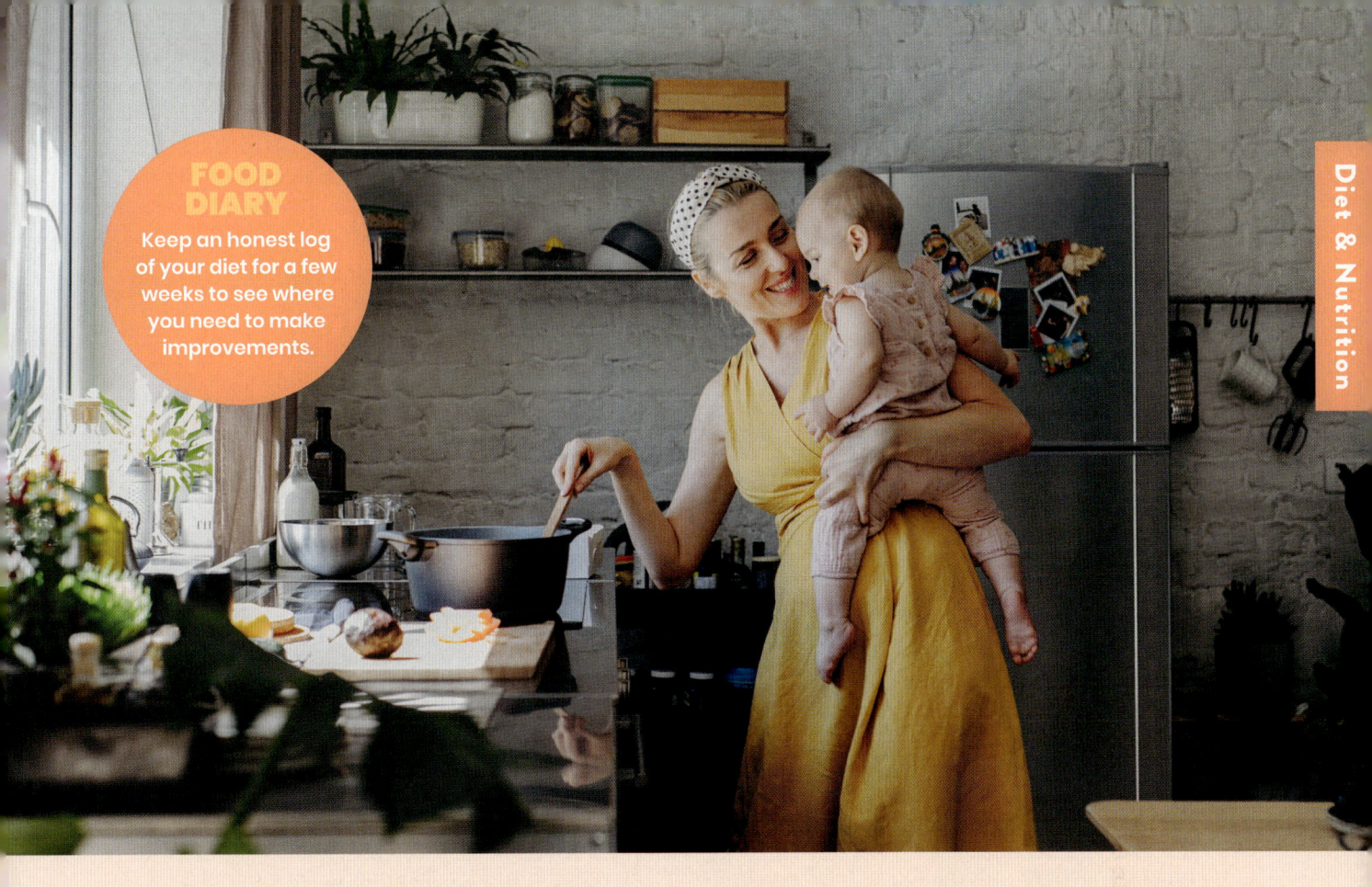

Keep an honest log of your diet for a few weeks to see where you need to make improvements.

sauces and canned fruit. A lot of added sugar comes from drinks, which is why it's best to stick to water where possible. While 'diet' versions of drinks don't have sugar in, they do have sweeteners, which give us that sweet taste and can increase cravings for more sugary foods.

> **"START SMALL – IT CAN BE HARD TO MAKE TOO MANY CHANGES AT ONCE"**

Salt is another big problem in our food. Having too much salt in your diet is one of the key factors in increasing blood pressure (hypertension), which can lead to stroke and heart failure. We do need a little salt in our diet, but adults should aim to have less than 6g of salt a day, which is about 1 level teaspoon. This includes the salt that is already in foods – the more processed a food is, the higher in salt it is likely to be.

Saturated fat raises cholesterol levels, and this can in turn increase your risk of heart disease. As a woman, you should aim to eat less than 20g of saturated fat a day. For context, one large glass of whole milk has about 7g of saturated fat. Saturated fat is found in fatty cuts of meat, butter, cheese, cream, biscuits, cakes and pastries.

Sugar, salt and saturated fat are all added to highly processed foods to make them taste good. If you eat too many ultraprocessed foods, it's likely that you are eating far too much of these substances. By switching to a less-processed diet, you will immediately lower your intake of these less-healthy foods and increase your intake of more healthy foods. A simple way to do this is to choose foods that don't have labels, because they are a single ingredient, such as an apple, or check food labels for items with ingredients that you recognise and you would find in a normal family kitchen.

HOW TO MAKE CHANGES TO YOUR DIET

When it comes to making positive changes to your diet, it's best to start small. It can be hard to make too many changes at once, especially if it marks a major change in the way you currently eat. It can be a good idea to keep a food diary for a couple of weeks to analyse your diet. Many of us under-report what we eat if we don't write it down. You might think your diet is broadly healthy, but a food diary can uncover trends and patterns that you haven't really considered.

You can do this simply in a notebook, but you might find it more helpful to use an app or digital tracker that will give you the nutritional breakdown of your weekly food intake. This can help you see in more detail what foods make up the bulk of your diet. Try not to think about one day at a time – aim instead to get a balance across a whole week.

Don't try to change everything at once – too many changes can make it harder to adhere to. Think about what you can add into your diet first, then consider what you might need to cut down or limit. Think of it as a long-term lifestyle change, not a short-term solution.

MENTAL HEALTH IN WOMEN

Manage your mental wellbeing and spot the signs of a problem

Looking after our mental health is just as important as looking after our physical health. The two are intrinsically linked – being in poor physical health can lead to mental-health conditions, just as struggling with our mental health can have physical symptoms too.

It's good to be aware of mental-health conditions and what the signs are, so that we're able to identify when we're not coping with life in the way that we usually would. Struggling with mental health is very common and can affect anyone of any sex and any age. However, there are some factors that can definitely increase the risk of mental-health issues.

COMMON CONDITIONS

One of the most common mental-health conditions is depression. We all have periods of low mood, stress, worry or anxiety, often triggered by a specific event. Depression is when we feel low and find it hard to enjoy life for a long time. There are different types of depression that vary in severity. Generalised depression is sometimes called major depressive disorder. Some people have a type of chronic depression called persistent depressive disorder (PDD), which is when the depression lasts for more than two years. Seasonal affective disorder (SAD) can impact some people at a particular time of year. It's best known for affecting people in the winter months, but SAD is not inherently a winter disorder. It's possible to have it in any season.

Other types of depression can be linked to certain hormonal disruptions. For example, antenatal depression is a type of depression that occurs during pregnancy; postnatal depression is depression that happens in the first year after having a baby; and premenstrual dysphoric disorder (PMDD) is something that can be linked to your menstrual cycle.

Anxiety is a common condition, especially among women. According to the Mental Health Foundation, women experience higher levels of anxiety than men, and younger women are more likely to have some form of anxiety than older women. Anxiety is when we feel stressed or worried about something that has happened or might happen. Everyone feels anxious sometimes and that's normal, but if you can't shake the feeling of worry and it's impacting on your daily life, this could be generalised anxiety disorder (GAD). Some people have particular types of anxiety, or a related disorder such as social anxiety, post-traumatic stress disorder (PTSD), obsessive-compulsive disorder (OCD), body dysmorphic disorder (BDD), health anxiety or a phobia.

Women are also three times more likely to develop an eating disorder than men, which includes anorexia, bulimia and binge eating. It's thought that more than a million people in the UK have an eating disorder.[1]

Anyone can develop a mental-health disorder, but there are some risk factors that can make it more likely. These factors can be social, economic, environmental or genetic. Women are more likely to be primary caregivers, whether that's for children or other relatives, which can be stressful and isolating (see the box on the next page for more). Women are also more likely to live in ▶

> "ANYONE CAN DEVELOP A MENTAL-HEALTH DISORDER, BUT THERE ARE RISK FACTORS THAT CAN MAKE IT MORE LIKELY"

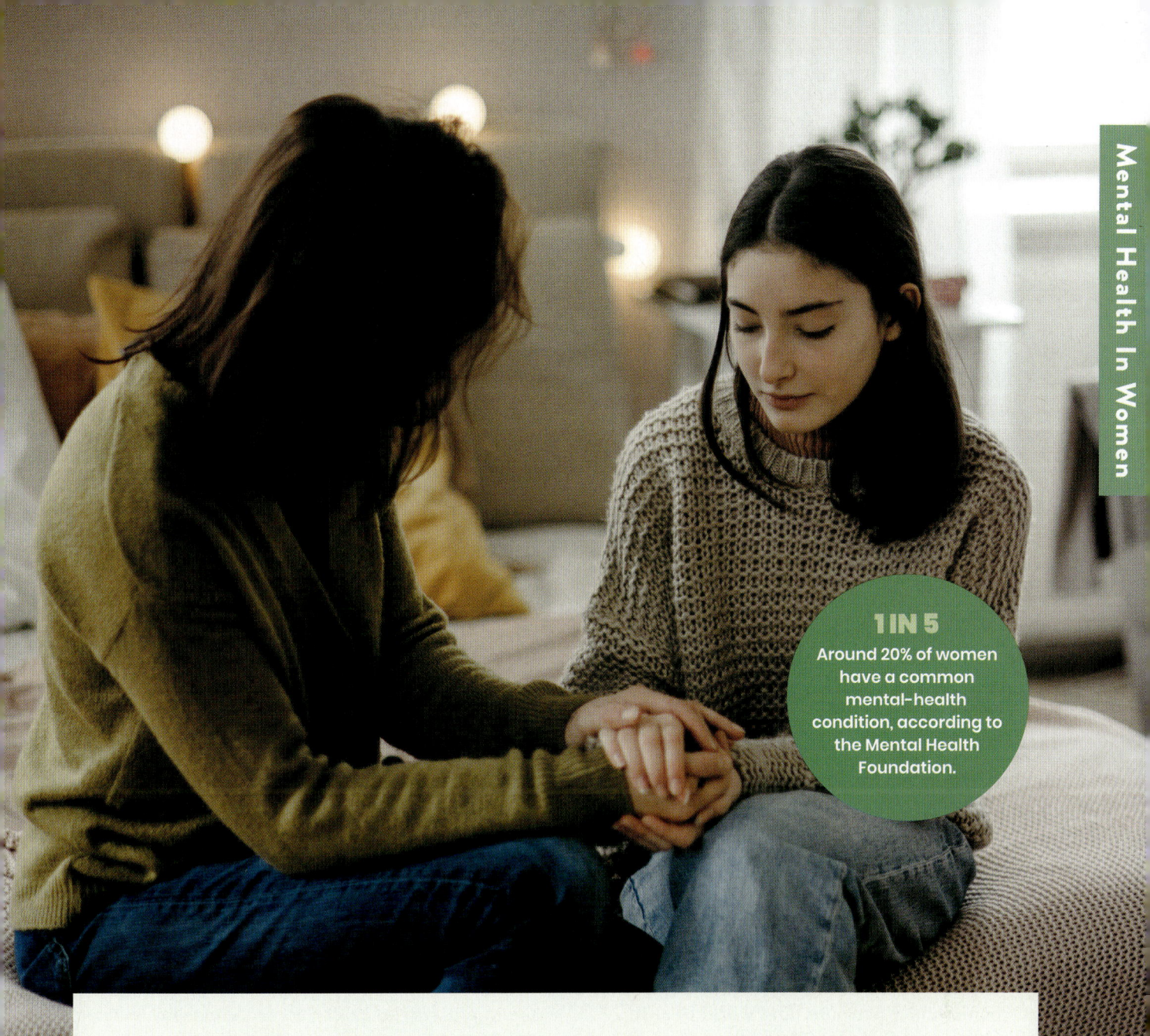

1 IN 5
Around 20% of women have a common mental-health condition, according to the Mental Health Foundation.

THE IMPACT OF CARING
RESPONSIBILITIES

Women often have additional caring duties that can affect their mental health

Whether you're a busy mother or caring for older parents, having to take on the responsibility of supporting others can be a significant factor when it comes to looking after your mental health. If you're guilty of constantly putting the needs of others above your own, your mental wellbeing could take a hit. Carers and parents often find that they don't get the time to exercise as much, cook healthy meals as often, or have time to do their own hobbies. It can be very stressful, especially if there is no respite. It's important to try to carve out some time to look after your own needs. If you're caring for a relative, you may be able to source some respite care for you to have a break. And if you're looking after young children, use whatever support you have around you to take time out. The more relaxed and stable you feel in yourself, the more you'll have to give to others.

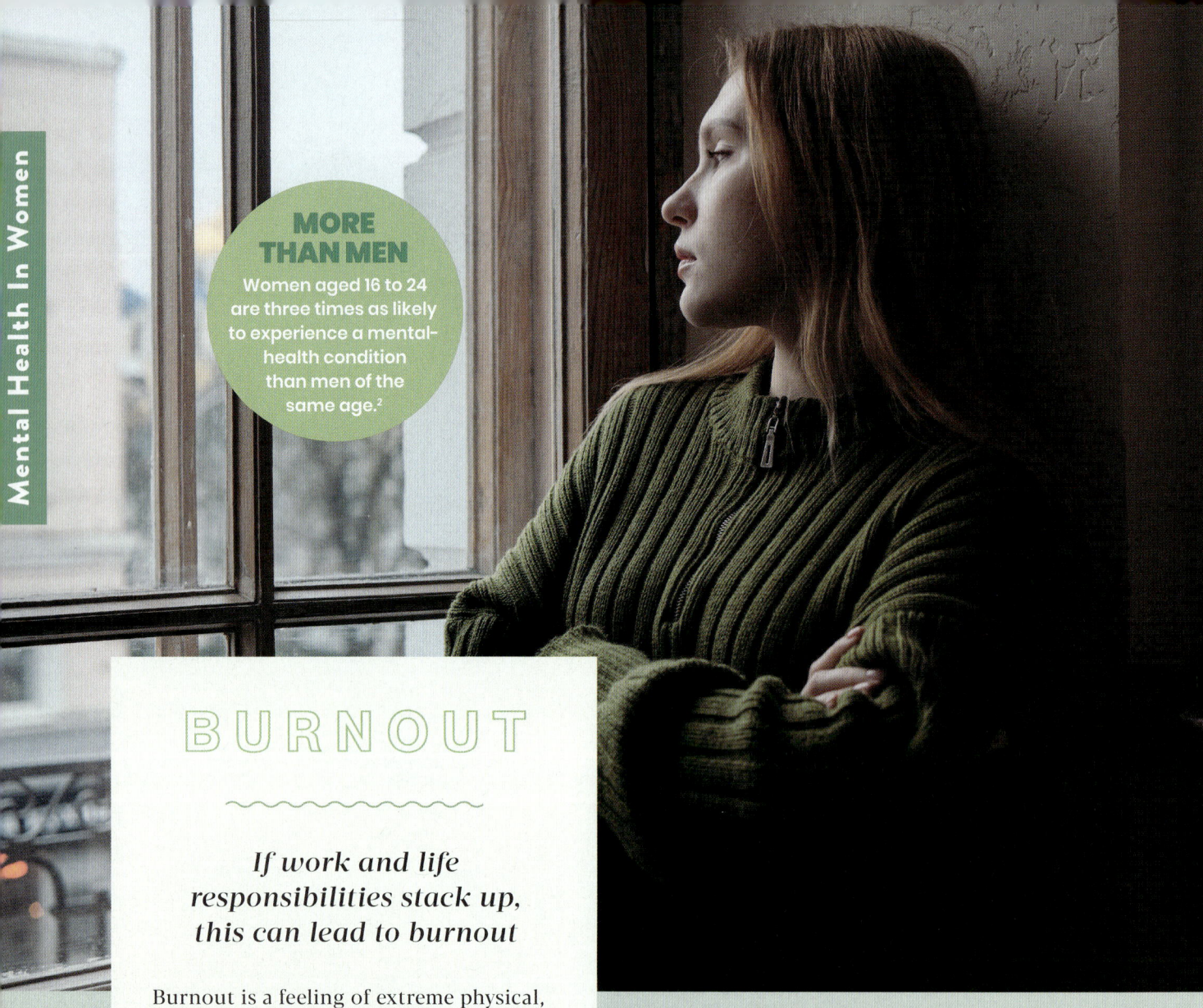

Mental Health In Women

MORE THAN MEN
Women aged 16 to 24 are three times as likely to experience a mental-health condition than men of the same age.[2]

BURNOUT

If work and life responsibilities stack up, this can lead to burnout

Burnout is a feeling of extreme physical, emotional and mental exhaustion, usually caused by long-term stress and being under pressure. The World Health Organization defines it as an 'occupational phenomenon' rather than a specific health condition, but it doesn't only happen to workers. It can come on suddenly, but the underlying causes have probably been there for a while. Burnout tends to affect women more than men, which may in part be due to societal expectations around juggling work life, home life and personal life. In Mental Health UK's 2025 Burnout Report, 94% of adult women reported that they have experienced high levels of stress in the past year. Symptoms can be physical, including feeling tired most of the time, joint pain, headaches, frequent illness, high blood pressure and insomnia. They can also be emotional, such as feeling hopeless, detached, overwhelmed or unable to enjoy everyday life. If any of this resonates, it's worth speaking to a doctor, as it often doesn't get better without some help.

▸ poverty, experience physical or sexual abuse, be under pressure to look or act a certain way, or have concerns around personal safety.

Hormonal changes in the body can also have an impact on our mental health. Puberty can affect the mental health of young girls, and low mood and increased anxiety are often associated with the onset of perimenopause.

SIGNS AND SYMPTOMS

It can sometimes be hard to spot the signs of a mental-health problem. Being self-aware and acknowledging your own thoughts and feelings can make it easier to spot when something is wrong, but not everyone is tuned in to their health in this way.

Mental-health conditions can impact on our mood, such as regular mood swings, prolonged periods of feeling sad or hopeless, feelings of inadequacy, finding it hard to be positive, and having obsessive or excessive worries and fears. Some people find it hard to focus, struggle with brain fog or feel paranoid. In more severe cases, someone might start to have thoughts around death or suicide.

Normal behaviour can also be disrupted. Many people with a mental-health issue will withdraw from their usual daily activities and stop seeing friends and family. Some may turn to alcohol or other forms of substance abuse to help cope with the way they're feeling, or they engage in high-risk activities. People with a mental-health condition can also find that their sex drive drops, they feel more angry than usual, or find it hard to control their thoughts and feelings.

Mental-health conditions can sometimes have physical symptoms too – such as fatigue, low energy levels, aches and pains, headaches, or digestive issues. These are all very generalised symptoms, as every mental-health issue presents differently. However, if you notice that you (or anyone you care for) is acting in a way that is out of character, it's time to seek professional advice. A mental-health condition is unlikely to resolve on its own, but early intervention can often help to treat the problem quickly.

> **"MANY PEOPLE WITH A MENTAL-HEALTH CONDITION WILL WITHDRAW AND STOP SEEING FRIENDS AND FAMILY"**

HELP FOR MENTAL HEALTH

If you already have signs and symptoms of a mental-health condition, then your doctor can advise you of the available treatment options. This can include talking therapies, like counselling or cognitive behavioural therapy (CBT), or even group sessions. You may also benefit from a course of medication that can help to restore some balance. These treatments are often used in conjunction with lifestyle changes and holistic practices; social prescribing is becoming a more popular way to treat common mental-health issues, and this can include anything from exercise groups to gardening.

We need to take a proactive approach and look after our mental health throughout our life in the same way that we look after our physical health. Good mental wellbeing helps us to live a fulfilling and happy life, but it also helps us to be more aware when we are struggling. With this in mind, you should find time to rest and relax every day – rest is good for both body and soul, and it's easy not to get enough of it. For some people, this might be sitting still and doing nothing; for others it might mean taking time to do something they enjoy, like reading a book, cooking or crafting. Being creative, in whatever way works for you, can also help with mental wellbeing. And our sleep is also a huge factor when it comes to mental health. Without good sleep, we're more prone to low moods and stress. We should all focus on creating a relaxing sleep environment, prioritising sleep quality and having a good bedtime routine.

Exercise can boost your mood and help to prevent depression and anxiety. Some people find that intense exercise, like running or team sports, can relieve stress and anxiety. Others find that mindful exercise, like yoga or Pilates, can balance the mind and body and help with relaxation. Being outside can also boost your mood, so try to combine exercise with nature by going for a walk or doing stretches in the garden.

Connection is another key area to focus on – we need our friends and family! Socialising, having people you can talk to, and connecting with others has been shown to have a positive impact on mental health. If you have a hobby or sport you enjoy, finding a group that enables you to take part with other people can help to tick off both exercise and social connection in one go.

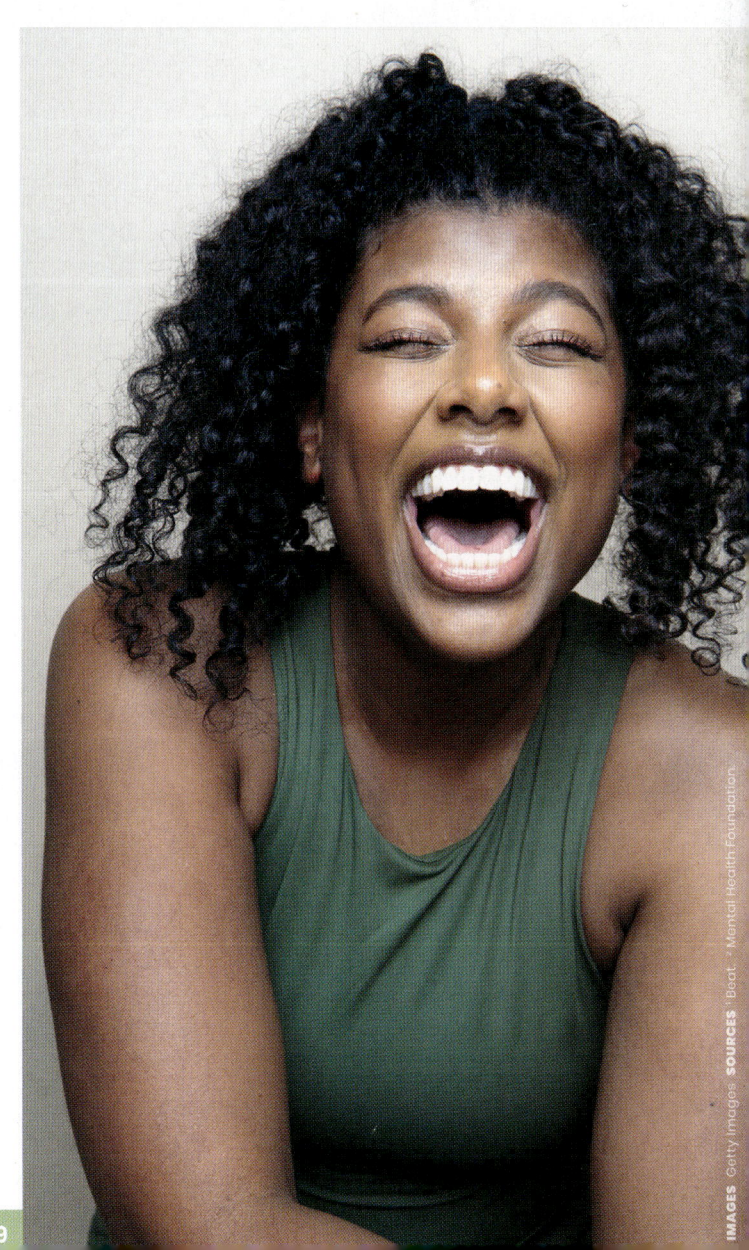

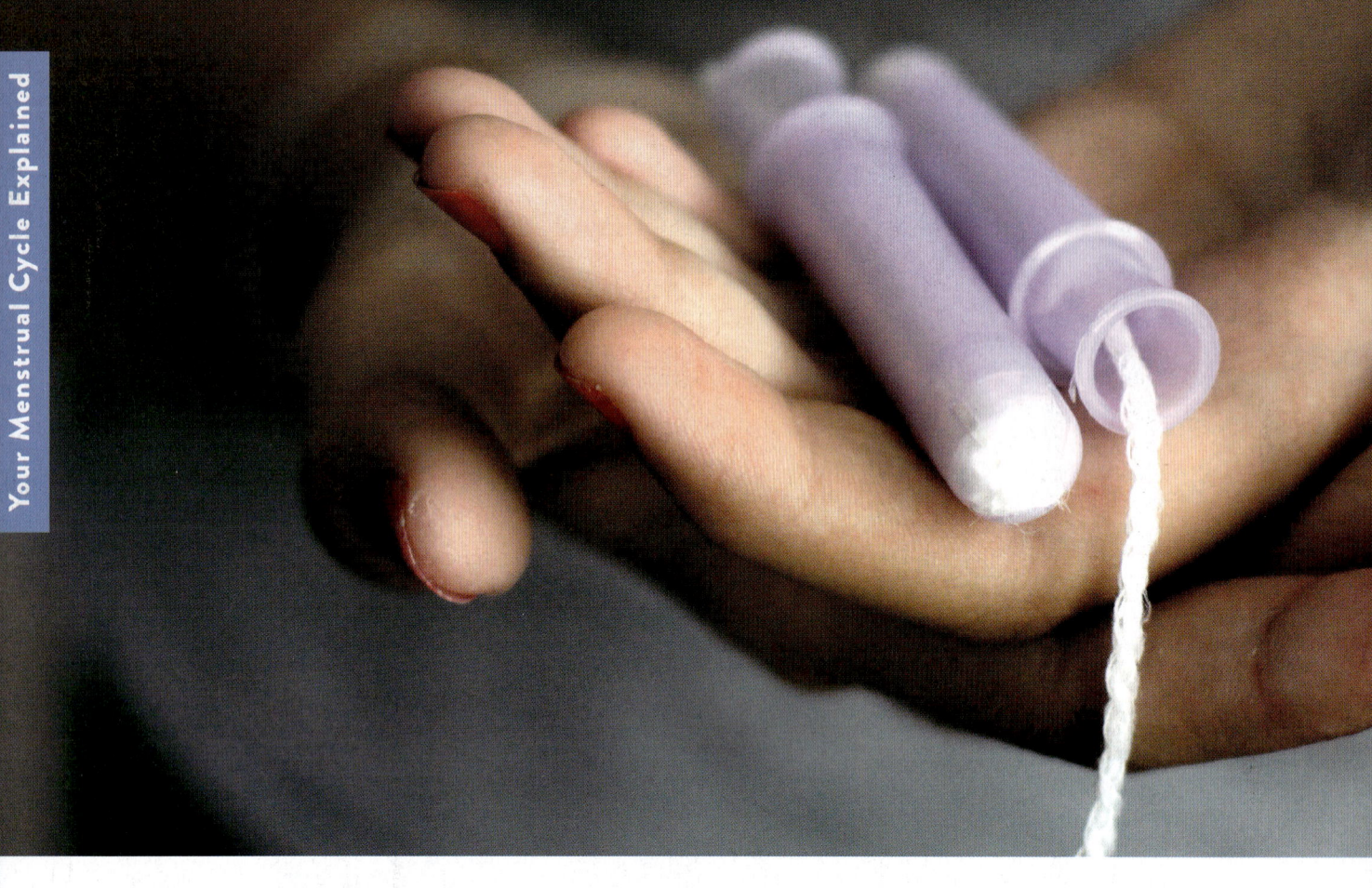

YOUR MENSTRUAL CYCLE EXPLAINED

It happens to most of us every month for decades, but what is actually going on inside our bodies?

A woman's menstrual cycle is the body's way of preparing for a possible pregnancy, adapting the body in lots of small ways through a (roughly) monthly cycle. It is broken down into four key stages, each of which changes the body in different ways. At puberty, a woman has on average of about 300,000 to 400,000 eggs, and that number depletes with each menstrual cycle.

In this feature, we will give you an overview of each of the four phases to understand what physical and emotional changes happen throughout a typical menstrual cycle. In the coming pages, we'll explore some of these phases in more detail.

PHASE 1: MENSTRUATION

The most obvious part of the menstrual cycle is menstruation (or menses), which is when you have your period. When an egg hasn't been fertilised, your hormone levels drop as they're not needed to support a pregnancy. This causes the body to shed the thickened uterine lining (endometrium), which passes out through the vagina. It takes, on average, three to seven days to be released from the body. The discharge that you see isn't just blood; it also contains mucus and tissue cells from the uterus.

During your period, you may suffer from various symptoms caused by your uterus contracting to

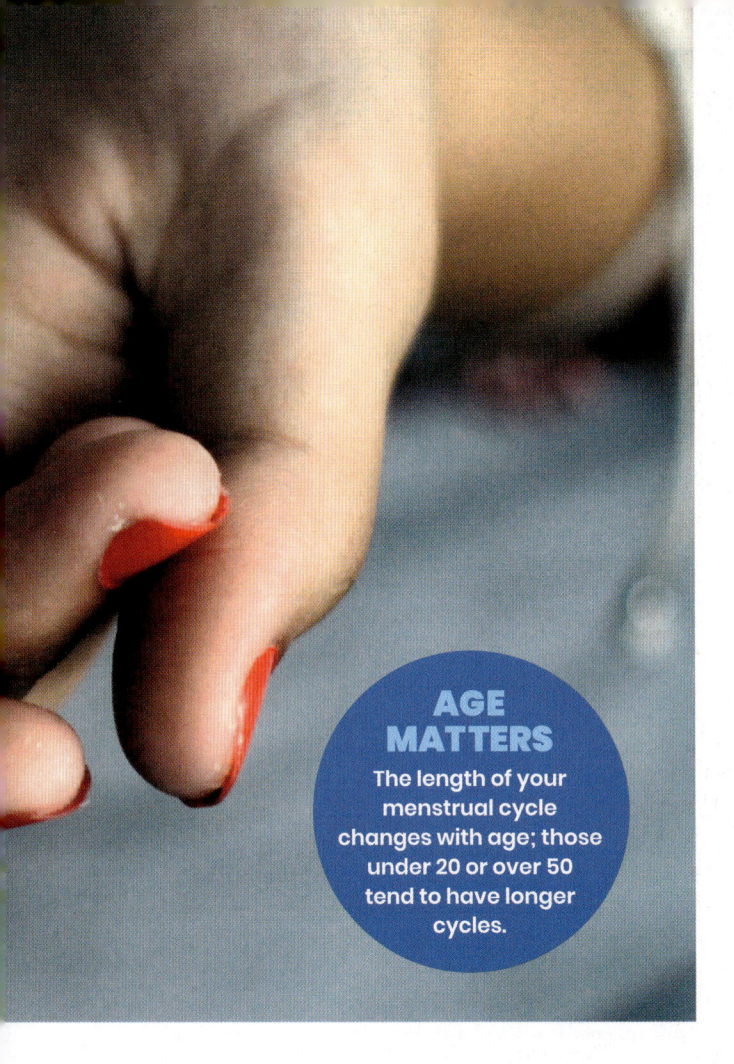

AGE MATTERS
The length of your menstrual cycle changes with age; those under 20 or over 50 tend to have longer cycles.

shed its lining, as well as directly due to your dropping hormone levels. These can include things like stomach cramps, tender or sore breasts, mood swings, bloating, feeling irritable or low, headaches, tiredness and lower back pain. Period symptoms are different for everyone, but there are treatments available to help relieve them. Periods themselves can vary a lot in terms of how much blood loss there is, how long they last and how they make you feel, but you will usually develop a sense of a pattern that's unique to you.

During your period you are at your least fertile, but it's not impossible to get pregnant at this time, so precautions should still be taken if you're not wanting to become pregnant. It can be more likely if you have irregular or short cycles. Sperm can survive for a few days, so if you ovulate shortly after your period and you've recently had unprotected penile-vaginal intercourse, then it is possible for an egg to be fertilised. Although unlikely, it's worth being aware of the possibility!

PHASE 2: FOLLICULAR

The follicular phase overlaps with menstruation, as it begins from the first day that your period starts and lasts until you ovulate. In a typical 28-day cycle, this means that the follicular stage can last for up to two weeks.

It's during this time that your hypothalamus sends a message to your pituitary gland to trigger the release of follicle-stimulating hormone (FSH).

PMS
& PMDD

Many women struggle with physical and emotional symptoms in the lead-up to their period

Pre-menstrual syndrome (PMS) is not uncommon but, depending on the severity of your symptoms, it can have a big impact on your day-to-day life in the days preceding the start of your period. It's thought that up to three in four women have PMS to some degree.[1] Quite a few of the symptoms are emotional, and this includes things like anxiety, low mood, irritability, restlessness, difficult focusing and increased appetite. It can also change sleep patterns. Women can experience physical symptoms including bloating, cramps, swollen breasts, skin problems, digestive issues and headaches. It's thought that PMS happens due to the hormonal changes in the body, but some lifestyle factors can make symptoms worse, including a poor diet, lack of exercise and smoking.

PMS symptoms that are more severe and have a huge impact on your life could be premenstrual dysphoric disorder (PMDD), which is recognised as a mental health condition and affects fewer than 5% of women.[1] Symptoms include depression, panic attacks, insomnia, sudden changes in mood and a loss of interest in normal activities. It's important to seek treatment, which can be a combination of medication, lifestyle changes and therapy.

The FSH's job is to stimulate your ovaries and develop follicles, which are sacs that each contain an immature egg. Multiple follicles develop for each cycle, the number of which is dependent on many factors, such as environment, health and age. From all these follicles, only one egg, usually the healthiest with the best chance of fertilisation, will be selected to mature. In rare cases, two eggs ▶

Your Menstrual Cycle Explained

PROMOTING A HEALTHY MENSTRUAL CYCLE

Having regular periods can influence our overall health

While a regular menstrual cycle is a sign of good health, being in good health also promotes a healthy menstrual cycle! If you are having regular periods with no significant issues, then your hormones are more balanced. Balanced hormones mean your moods are likely more stable, and you have more consistent energy levels. If you have steady hormone levels, you may also be less prone to some of the physical symptoms of the menstrual cycle, like bloating and cramps. Oestrogen is also important for immune function, so having a regular cycle can mean that you're less likely to get ill and you may recover more quickly when you get an infection. Having an irregular cycle can often be a sign of an underlying issue. This is why lifestyle factors are key for so many different areas of our health. Eating well, drinking plenty of water, not smoking or drinking too much alcohol, getting enough sleep and maintaining a healthy weight all help to ensure your menstrual cycle functions optimally for you.

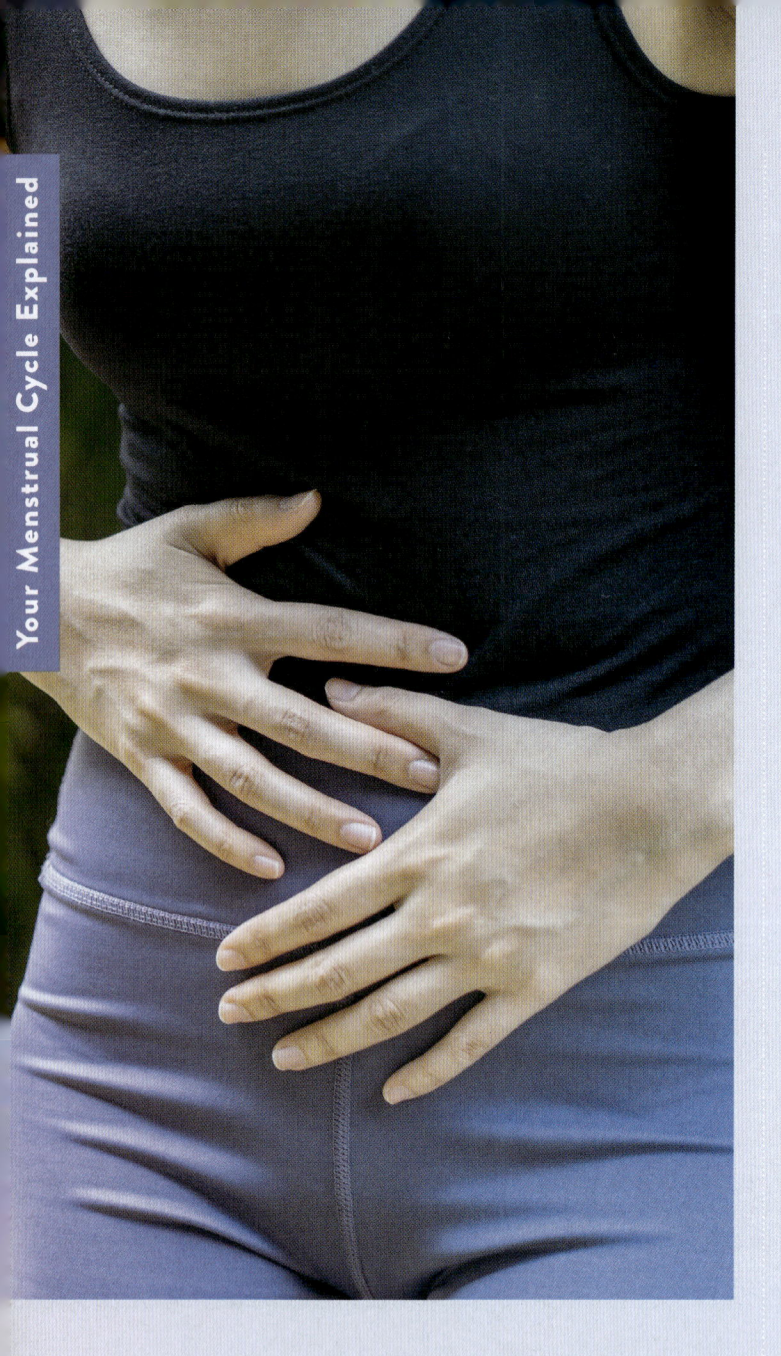

▶ might mature in a process called hyperovulation, both with the potential to be fertilised, which can then lead to fraternal, or non-identical, twins being conceived. Any remaining follicles that are not matured are reabsorbed into the body.

The process of maturing an egg within a follicle triggers the release of oestrogen, so that your hormone levels begin to rise to help develop the optimal conditions for an embryo to thrive. During the follicular phase, your fertility also begins to increase. From the middle of this phase through to the start of ovulation, it is possible to conceive, peaking at the end of the follicular phase, during ovulation and just after ovulation.

PHASE 3: OVULATION

At the end of your follicular phase, the rise in oestrogen levels sends another message to your pituitary gland, this time telling it to release the luteinising hormone (LH). This triggers the release of the mature egg by opening the follicle. The egg is then moved down the fallopian tubes through muscle contractions towards the uterus. Here the egg is ready to potentially be fertilised by sperm. This is when you are at your most fertile and therefore most likely to get pregnant. Usually this happens in the middle of your menstrual cycle, so around day 14 in a typical 28-day cycle. Ovulation only lasts for about a day, when the egg is viable. After this time, the egg will either be fertilised, in which case it will continue on towards the uterus and implant into its lining, or it won't and the egg will die and dissolve.

Many women are aware of when they ovulate due to feeling certain symptoms. The most common sign is a white vaginal discharge that is thicker than usual, as well as possibly cramps due to the muscle contractions. There is often a rise in basal body temperature, which is your body's lowest temperature at rest. Some people track their basal body temperature to help predict when they are at their most fertile, whether for the purposes of conceiving a baby or to practise a form of natural contraception. (We have more on this in our features on conception and contraception later.)

During ovulation, you may find that your sex drive increases, a natural bodily response linked to your heightened state of fertility. You might also have mood swings and anxiety around this time.

PHASE 4: LUTEAL

The final phase is the luteal phase, which overlaps with ovulation and lasts for an average of 14 days. It starts after the egg has been released from the follicle and started its journey towards the uterus. At this point, the follicle that housed the egg changes into a temporary gland called the 'corpus luteum'. Its role is to produce progesterone, which helps to thicken the lining of the uterus for potential implantation of a fertilised egg. If fertilisation is successful, the corpus luteum remains, producing hormones that are required to help the pregnancy progress. Otherwise, it breaks down and is reabsorbed by the body.

This process is what starts to lower your hormone levels. As your levels start to drop off, it triggers the shedding of the uterine lining and brings you back round to menstruation. It's during this phase that you might experience premenstrual syndrome (PMS) – see the box on page 51 on this – which can impact a woman up until their period starts. If you get pregnant during this time, then you won't progress to menstruation and your menstrual cycles will pause.

> **"DURING OVULATION, YOU MAY FIND THAT YOUR SEX DRIVE INCREASES"**

Understanding what a normal, healthy menstrual cycle should be like can help you to identify when something isn't right. However, there are many things that can disrupt the cycle, including your health, any underlying conditions and whether you use hormonal contraception. You need to learn what's normal for you and seek medical advice if you notice any changes.

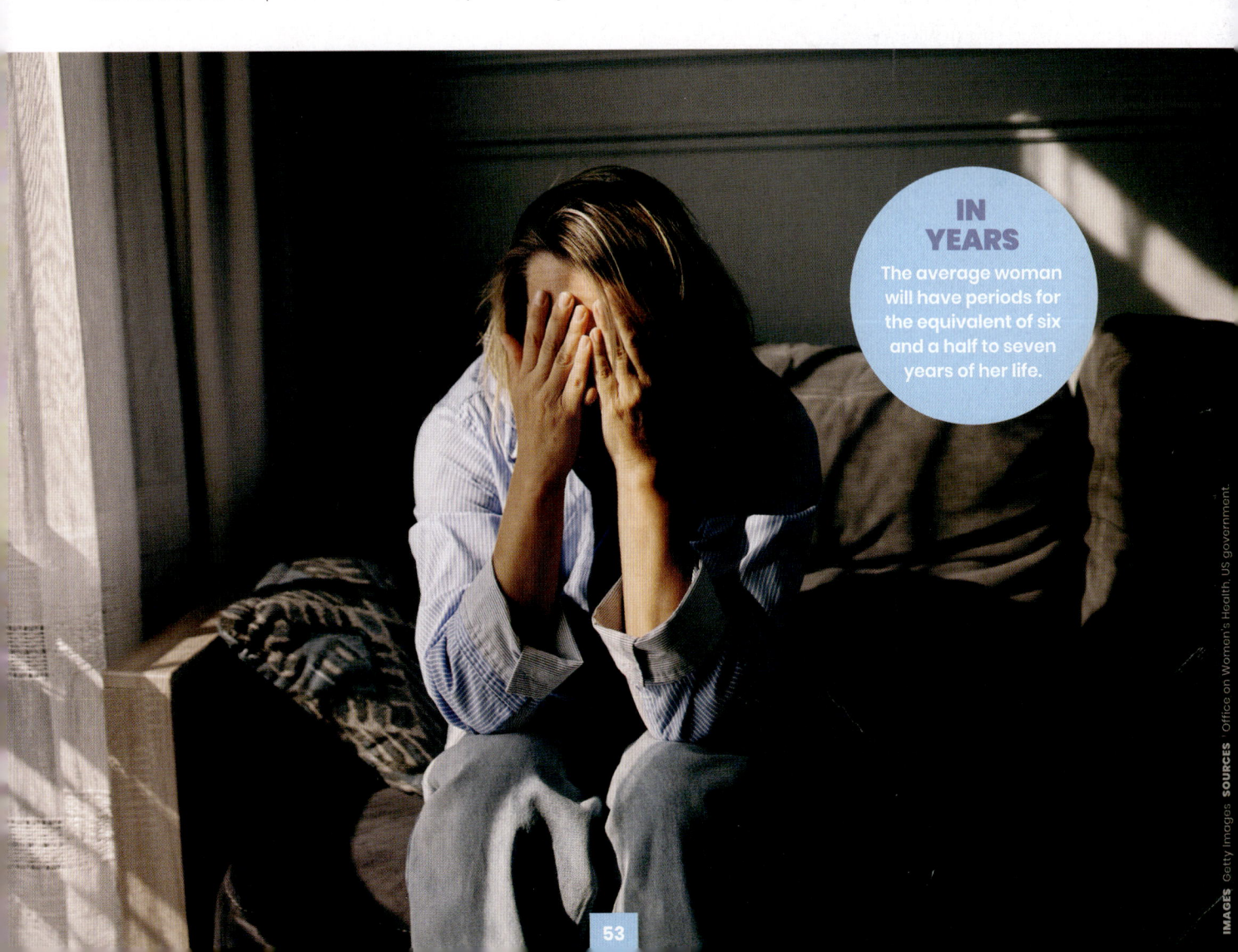

IN YEARS
The average woman will have periods for the equivalent of six and a half to seven years of her life.

A Guide To Periods

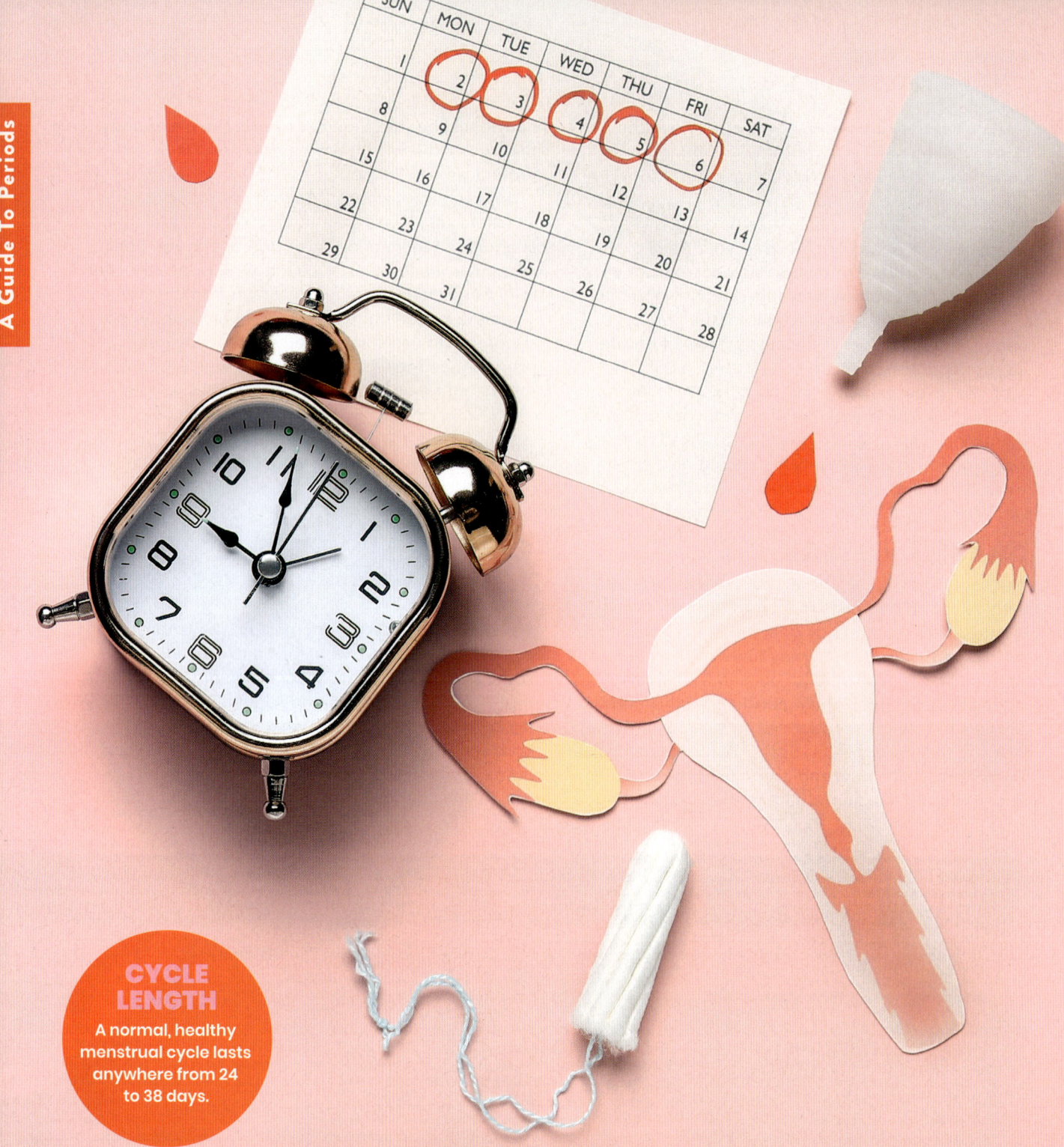

CYCLE LENGTH
A normal, healthy menstrual cycle lasts anywhere from 24 to 38 days.

A GUIDE TO
PERIODS

Everything you need to know about healthy periods and common period problems

For most of your teenage and adult life, periods will be something you have to think about. You might worry about starting them and ending them. You might panic when they come on unexpectedly, and worry when they don't come at all. They might be a fact of life, but that doesn't stop them from being a nuisance at times and something we have to plan around as women.

In order to know when periods are a problem, it's important to know what a healthy period looks and feels like. We've already discussed the menstrual cycle and what is happening inside your body in terms of reproductive processes and hormones in the previous pages. But here we will find out more about things like colour, smell, flow, volume and pain. It might not be pleasant to think about, but learning 'your normal' can be important for body awareness.

HEALTHY PERIODS

Period blood isn't always bright red; it varies depending on where you are in your cycle. Any variation of red, pink, brown or even black can be normal, but it's good to be aware of the signs that something isn't quite right. You may notice that you have a pinky discharge right before your period, where small amounts of blood are mixing into your normal discharge. It's often a sign that your period is imminent. You might then get bright-red, fresh blood at the start of your period as your uterus quickly starts to shed its lining. Over time, it may begin to darken in colour, which is completely normal. The uterus will contract slower and shed the lining less quickly, meaning that the blood is less fresh and therefore darker. Older blood that has been outside the blood vessels for longer can be brown in colour – or even black – and again, that's not unusual. This is simply due to the oxidisation process when the blood mixes with oxygen in the air.

Over time you'll learn what a healthy colour range is for you, which means that if you spot something different, you can see your doctor to get a check-up. Things to watch out for include orange- or grey-coloured discharge, especially if accompanied by any itching, strong smell, pain or discomfort, as these could be signs of an infection. And if you're pregnant, any colour in your discharge should always be checked out.

ALL ABOUT FLOW

As well as colour, your flow rate and blood loss may vary. On average, a woman will lose anywhere from 20-90ml of blood per period, which is equivalent to about 1-5 tablespoons. It's normal to have a lighter flow at the beginning and end of a period, and then a couple of heavier days in the middle. You may also notice clots of blood, normally no bigger than a coin, which can be tissue from the uterus. They can be more common at the beginning of your period and can vary in colour depending on how fresh the blood is. If the clots are large or it's painful to pass them, that is definitely something that needs to be looked at.

Some women struggle with extra heavy periods (known as menorrhagia), and this can have a significant impact on their life. A heavy period is defined as losing more than 80ml of blood per period or bleeding for longer than a week. It can

> "IT'S IMPORTANT TO KNOW WHAT A HEALTHY PERIOD LOOKS LIKE"

TRACKING YOUR PERIODS

The best way to spot problems is to keep track

If you don't already, then it's worth keeping track of your periods in some way. This makes it much easier to determine when something changes. It doesn't matter how you track your cycle – it just needs to be something you'll keep up with. Some people prefer to have a manual method, marking it down on a calendar or in a diary. It only needs to have the first day of your period and the last, but you may want to add more details.

There are period-tracking apps where you can log things like your flow, blood colour and symptoms to help build up a bigger picture of your menstrual health. It can be particularly useful for those who are looking to conceive, as it can help to identify your most fertile window, as well as those who might be coming close to perimenopause when periods can become more irregular.

> **"MANY WOMEN FIND THAT APPLYING HEAT CAN HELP, AS IT RELAXES MUSCLES"**

be hard to measure volume by eye, so it's easier to keep track of how often you need to change your period products. If you need to change your pad or tampon at least every three hours on your worst days, or you need to use both a tampon and a pad to prevent leaks, you may be passing more blood than expected. Some women also find that they regularly bleed through onto clothes or in bed.

There are treatment options depending on what the underlying cause is. Some possible causes could be fibroids, polycystic ovary syndrome (PCOS), adenomyosis, endometriosis, an infection, a health condition like an underactive thyroid, or in the worst case it can be a sign of cancer.

However, there may be no underlying cause at all – some women simply have heavier periods than others. It's more normal to have heavier periods when you are first starting your periods in puberty, and when you're approaching menopause. In any case, you should consult with a doctor, as blood loss can lead to iron deficiency (anaemia), and you may need to take supplements to combat this.

COPING WITH PAIN

Many women have some degree of pain when they have their period. It's not uncommon, and for most women it is relatively mild and resolved with painkillers. However, for others the pain can be far more severe and have a huge impact on day-to-day life.

Painful periods (called dysmenorrhoea) can be either primary or secondary. Primary dysmenorrhoea is period pain with no underlying cause, whereas secondary dysmenorrhoea is when it's caused by a health condition like endometriosis, the most common cause, or fibroids. While the pain is usually felt most in the abdomen, it can also spread to the back and the tops of the legs.

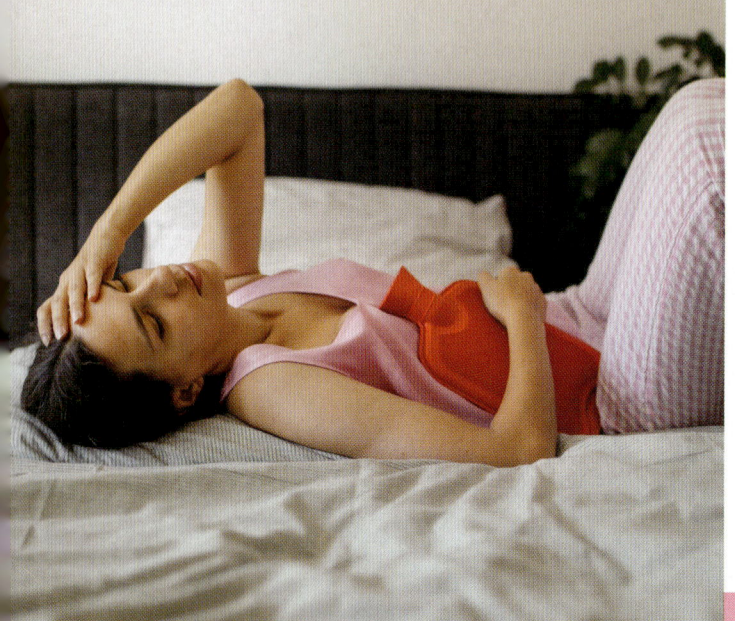

Whether you have a little pain or a lot, you may need to build up a toolkit to help you cope, especially if it's impacting your day. Over-the-counter painkillers can help with the pain, but if you are finding that they're not enough, your doctor may be able to prescribe something a little stronger. Many women find that applying heat can help, as it relaxes the muscles and relieves the pain. You could use a heat patch or a hot water bottle, or relax in a warm bath. Sometimes exercise can be beneficial too; you might not feel up to anything too intense, but stretching, yoga or walking can all be effective. You may also want to experiment with period products, as sometimes changing from tampons to pads, for example, can help.

OTHER PROBLEMS WITH PERIODS

Irregular periods are quite common. They are defined as being irregular when the length of time between periods is less than 21 days or more than 35 days. We all have irregular periods from time to time. It is more common during puberty, when your cycle is starting to establish itself, and towards menopause age when your hormone levels are beginning to decline. It's a good idea to track your periods (see the box on the previous page) to help determine what's normal for you and to identify any change in pattern.

Sometimes there is an underlying reason for irregular periods, or even skipping a period, such as PCOS or an underactive thyroid, but your cycle can be disrupted in other ways. If you lose or gain a lot of weight, this can impact your periods, as can higher levels of stress, anxiety or physical exertion. Absent periods (called amenorrhea), which last for three months or more, are often caused by a hormonal imbalance, if pregnancy is ruled out. It's worth seeing a doctor if your periods suddenly stop and you're not pregnant or at the usual age for menopause.

It can be hard to know when to see a doctor, but you should always go for a check-up if:

- Your periods last for over a week
- Your periods are changing in pattern or flow
- Your periods are becoming less frequent
- You have severe pain or flow that affects your daily life
- You notice blood between periods
- You see blood after having sex

You know your body best, so if something doesn't feel right, it's always better to get checked out.

A Guide To Periods

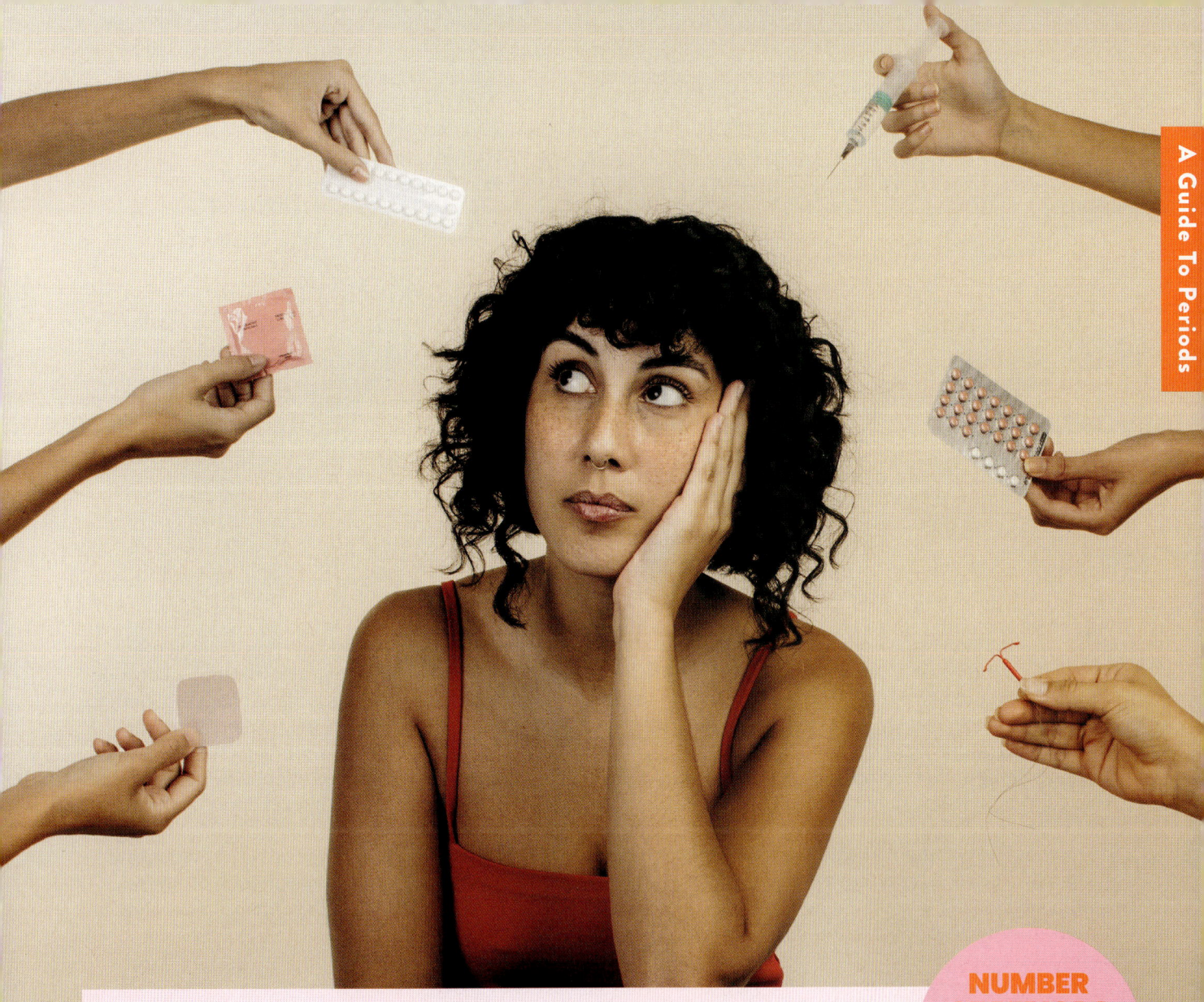

PERIODS & CONTRACEPTION

NUMBER OF PERIODS
The average woman will have around 450 to 500 periods over a lifetime.

You won't experience periods in the same way if you are using hormonal contraception

The type of contraception that you use can impact on your periods, and in some cases are used specifically to help with period problems. If you have painful periods, you may be advised to try hormonal contraception, such as the combined pill, hormonal coil, implant or injection, which can help to relieve pain. Similarly, these forms of contraception can help to reduce heavy periods. However, if you have the non-hormonal copper coil (IUD), you may experience heavier and more painful periods in the first few months.

When you have hormonal contraceptives, you won't always have a natural period. For example, if you use the combined pill, you will normally have regular bleeds because you have a break from the hormones each month and your body has a withdrawal bleed that is similar to a period. The contraceptive implant can change your periods too, making them either stop completely, lighter, more irregular or even heavier. It can take a bit of trial and error to work out what's best for your body.

WHAT IMPACTS OVULATION

There are many factors that can influence your ability to ovulate

Ovulation is the key part of the menstrual cycle when it comes to reproduction. The production of high-quality, mature eggs is what retains our fertility. Fertility works on a curve; we're not equally fertile from the moment our periods start until the day we have our last period. Our egg quality and quantity naturally decline with age.

Some time between our late teenage years and late 20s, we reach peak fertility, which is when we have the best chances of conceiving in any menstrual cycle. Of course, this is just when our body is at its peak fertility, and doesn't indicate when we're actually ready to have a baby. Between these ages you have about a 25% chance of getting pregnant in any given monthly cycle. From your early 30s, even though you are likely still ovulating every month, your chances of conceiving as a result are starting to decline, with a 10% chance of getting pregnant in any given monthly cycle after the age of 35. That drops much lower as we get older, and for most people, by the time we reach 50, the ovaries are depleted and the chance of pregnancy is almost non-existent.

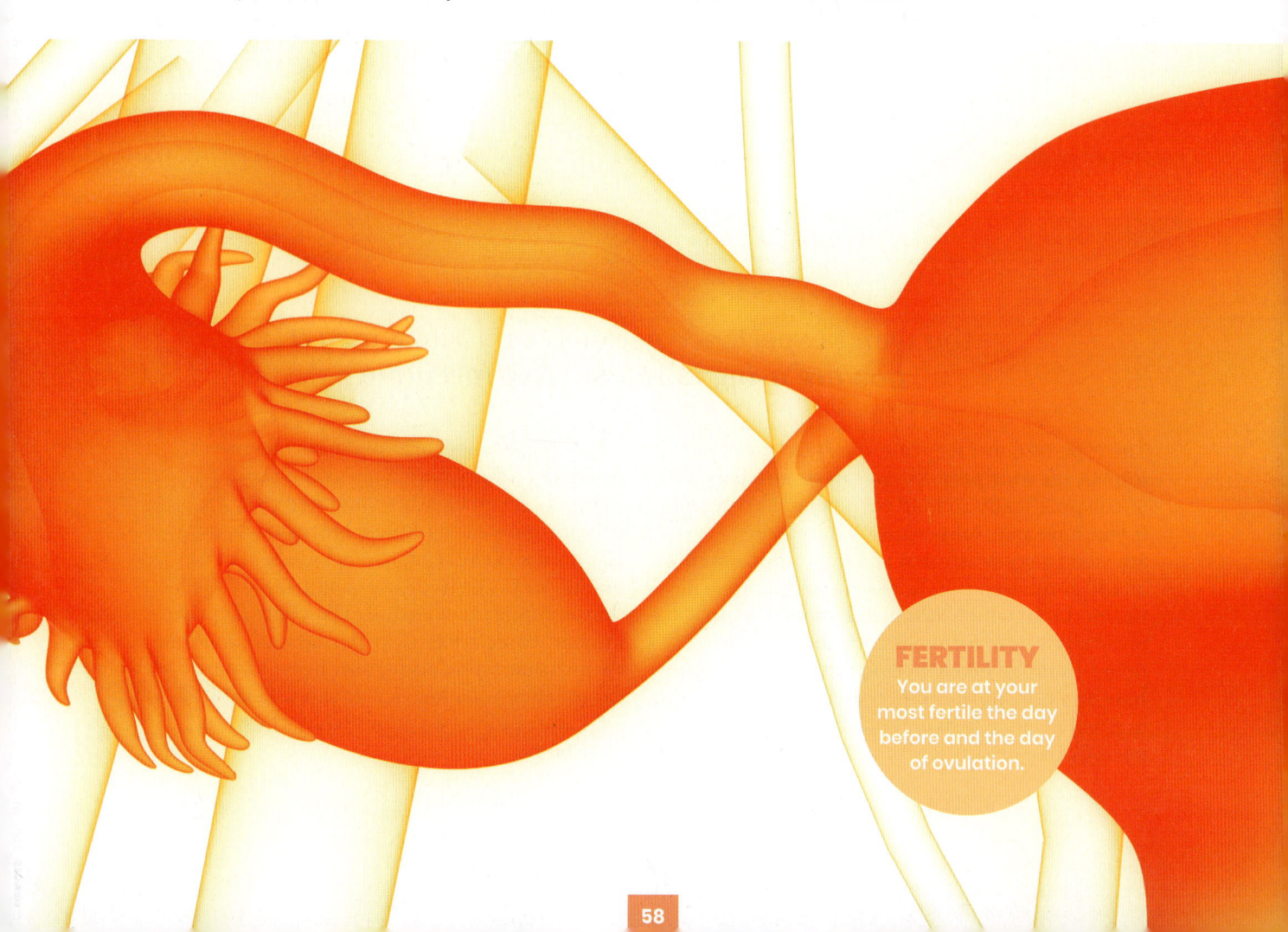

FERTILITY
You are at your most fertile the day before and the day of ovulation.

FACTORS THAT INFLUENCE OVULATION

Age is, therefore, one of the biggest factors that influences ovulation, but there are other things that can have an impact. Some of these are medical conditions and some are lifestyle factors; some are modifiable, while others are not.

Your body weight can affect ovulation. Being overweight can be a cause of irregular periods, which means that the body is not ovulating every month as it should. Women who are overweight can take longer to get pregnant in comparison to women of a healthy weight, even if they do have a regular cycle. Being underweight can also influence ovulation, particularly in women who have a body mass index (BMI) of under 19. In some cases, the body may stop producing an egg each month, causing irregular periods.

Your diet, whether you smoke, how much alcohol you drink and the exercise you do can also have an impact on your body's ability to ovulate optimally. If you're taking hormonal contraceptives, then these will prevent ovulation from taking place, so no egg will be released.

Health conditions that can cause problems with ovulation include things like an underactive or overactive thyroid or PCOS, both of which can imbalance hormone levels. Some medications may cause prolactin levels to rise (hyperprolactinemia), which prevents normal ovulation, and some treatments for other conditions, like certain cancers, can damage the ovaries and may cease ovulation.

When you're under a lot of stress, your body may shut down ovulation temporarily. It's thought that having more cortisol in the system, released by the body when it's in fight-or-flight mode, interrupts the usual balance of the female sex hormones. Stress doesn't just mean anxiety and worry; you can stress your body in other ways. Some people who undertake intense sport, for example training to run a marathon, may find that their body ceases ovulating due to the additional strain on the body.

If you're not ovulating, then it's usually a sign that something isn't right in your body, and a warning sign to speak to a doctor to find out more.

> **"DIET, SMOKING, ALCOHOL AND HOW MUCH EXERCISE YOU DO CAN HAVE AN IMPACT ON YOUR BODY'S ABILITY TO OVULATE"**

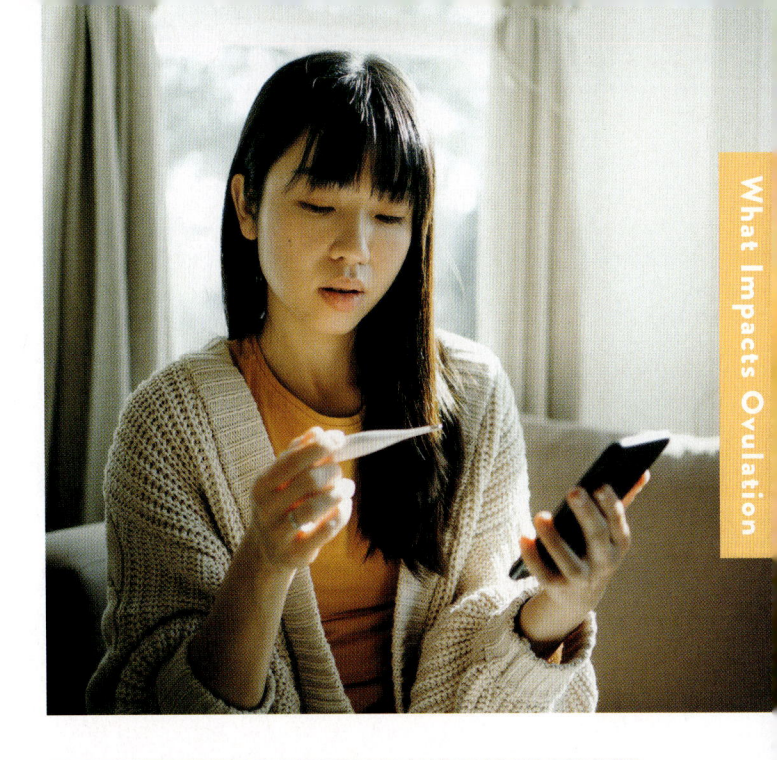

DETECTING OVULATION

There are various methods you can use to determine when you're ovulating

Many women track their ovulation for various reasons, but most commonly when they're looking to conceive. You can buy ovulation testing kits, similar to a pregnancy test, that detect hormone levels in your urine. They are looking at the luteinising hormone (LH), which tends to rise in the day or so before you ovulate. But you don't need to invest in kits if you're in tune with your body. If you're tracking your period, you may be able to pinpoint where in your cycle you ovulate, particularly if you are keeping track of your symptoms. You may notice, for example, a change in your cervical mucus, which can become clear and looser during ovulation, or minor pain in your pelvis or abdomen when the egg is released. Some women also track their basal body temperature using a thermometer that can detect minute changes. Many normal daily activities can raise your basal temperature, so it's important to follow the instructions to get an accurate reading.

CONTRACEPTION
OPTIONS

A quick guide to common contraceptives and how they work

CONTRACEPTIVE INJECTION

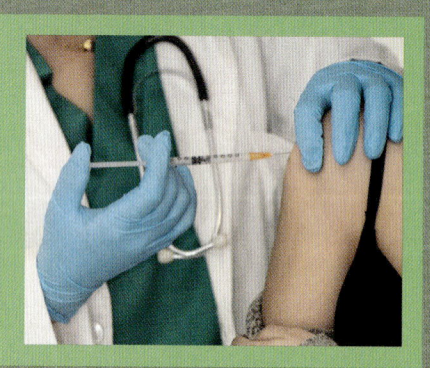

This injection contains progestogen, which prevents ovulation. It is over 99% effective against pregnancy, as long as the injection schedule is adhered to. Each injection lasts from 8 to 13 weeks, depending on the type of injection you have. It can take longer for your fertility to return to normal after stopping the injection than other forms of contraception – up to a year.

MALE CONDOMS

This is one of the most common forms of contraception. A condom is worn by a man on his penis, preventing any sperm from entering the vagina, meaning that fertilisation can't take place. They are also effective at preventing sexually transmitted infections, so they're often used alongside other hormonal contraceptive methods. If used properly and carefully, they can be up to 98% effective at preventing pregnancy; but when used incorrectly, the effectiveness can drop to 82%.

FEMALE CONDOMS

Female condoms are inserted into the vagina as far as possible, with an outer ring that remains external. They help to protect against pregnancy as well as sexually transmitted infections. If used properly and carefully, they can be up to 95% effective at preventing pregnancy; but when used incorrectly, the effectiveness can drop to 79%. They are not used as commonly as male condoms.

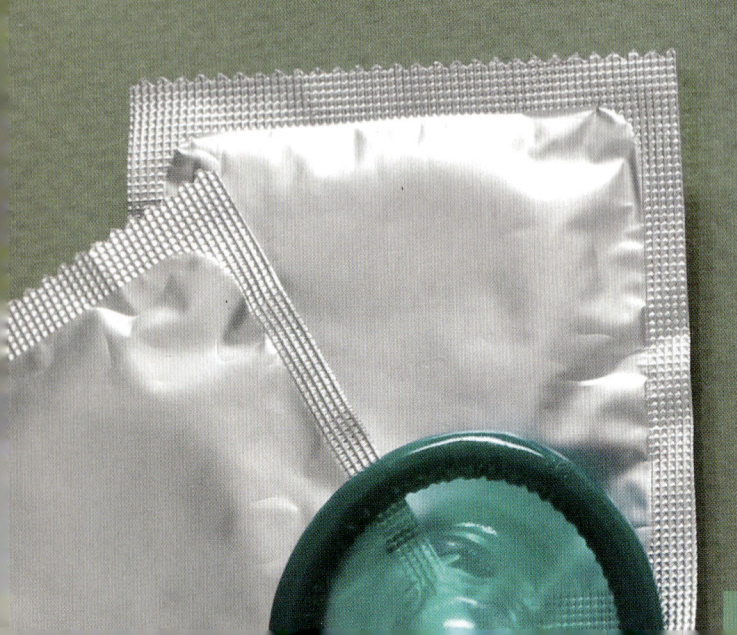

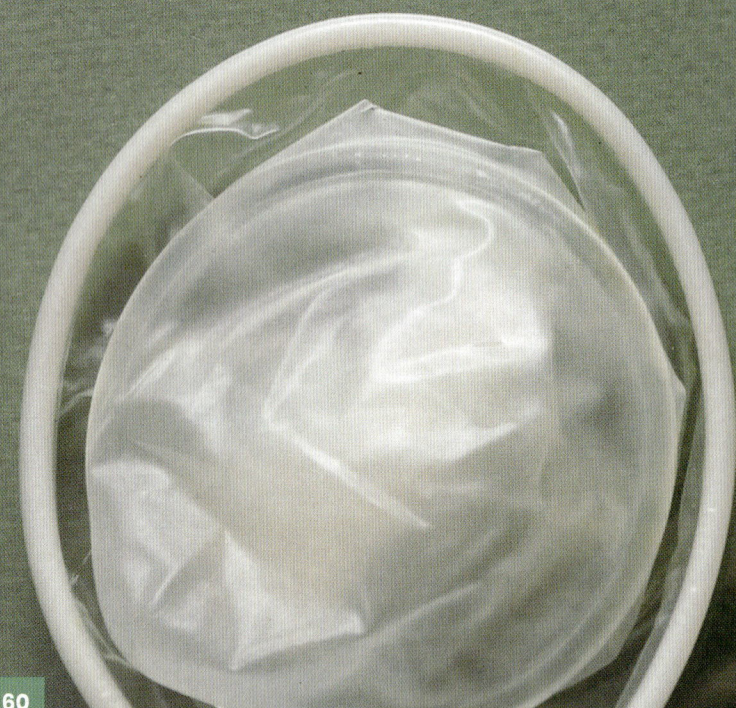

MINI PILL

The progestogen-only pill, or mini pill, acts in a similar way to the progesterone we naturally produce in our bodies. It prevents the ovaries from releasing an egg and is 99% effective against pregnancy. It can sometimes be suitable for those who can't take the combined pill, but there are still some for whom it might not be the right choice, such as those with cardiovascular disease or a liver condition.

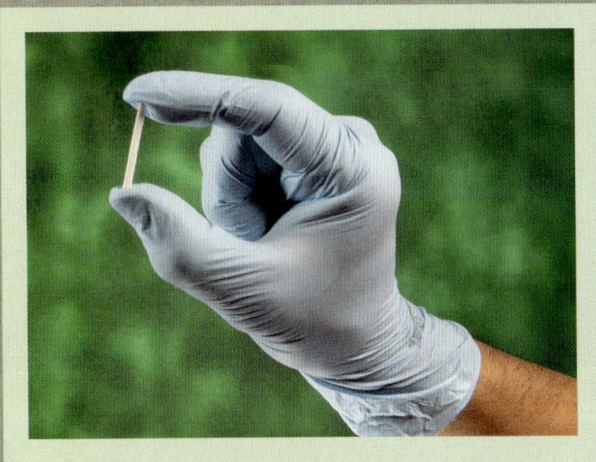

CONTRACEPTIVE IMPLANT

This is a small plastic pellet that is placed under the skin in your arm. It releases progestogen into your body, preventing the ovaries from releasing an egg. One benefit of the implant is that it lasts for three years before it's replaced, meaning you don't need to remember to take a pill every day. After three years it is less effective, but as long as you keep on top of it, it is over 99% effective.

HORMONAL COIL

An intrauterine system (IUS) is a hormonal device shaped like a 'T' that is placed into your uterus. It releases progestogen, preventing ovulation. It can last for three to eight years and is 99% effective at preventing pregnancy. Some people use it as a treatment for heavy periods, or to help with some menopause symptoms. It's important to note that using a coil does not protect against sexually transmitted infections.

COMBINED PILL

The combined contraceptive pill has both oestrogen and progestogen, which work together to stop the ovaries from releasing an egg. It is 99% effective against pregnancy, as long as it is used properly. It does not protect against sexually transmitted infections. Not everyone can tolerate the combined pill, and there are some people who are advised not to take it, such as those with a history of blood clots or certain cancers, and those with some existing health conditions.

COPPER COIL

An intrauterine device (or IUD), sometimes called the copper coil, is a non-hormonal form of contraception. It looks like a plastic 'T' and is placed into your uterus by a doctor or nurse. It releases copper into the womb, preventing pregnancy, and is 99% effective. It can last five to ten years, meaning you don't have to remember a pill every day, and fertility returns to normal as soon as it's removed. It can be a good option for those who can't use hormonal contraceptive options.

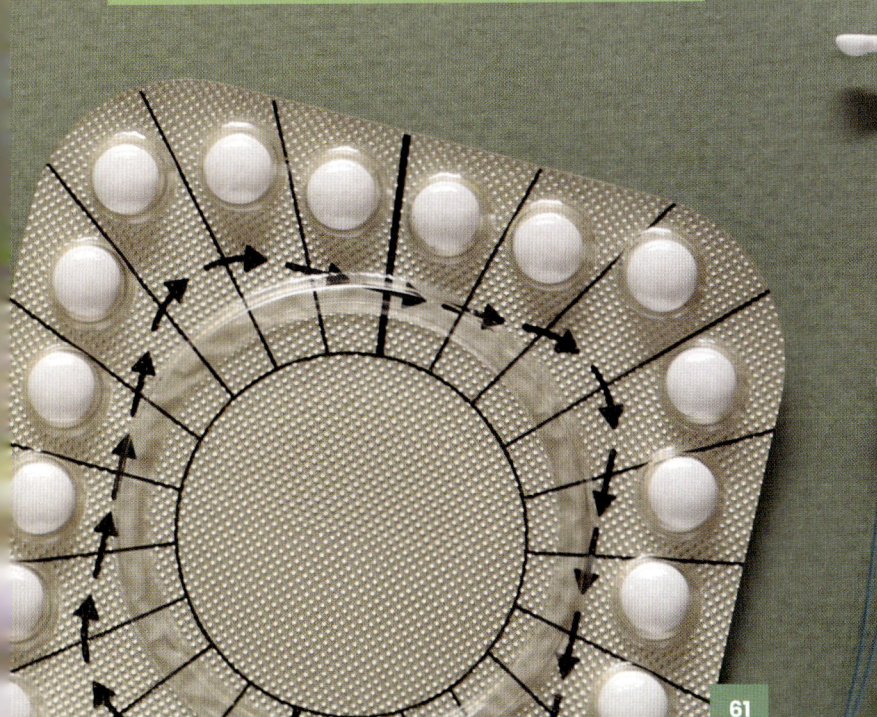

MOST COMMON

The most used forms of contraception are the male condom and the contraceptive pill.

UNDERSTANDING CONCEPTION

Everything you need to know about the process of getting pregnant

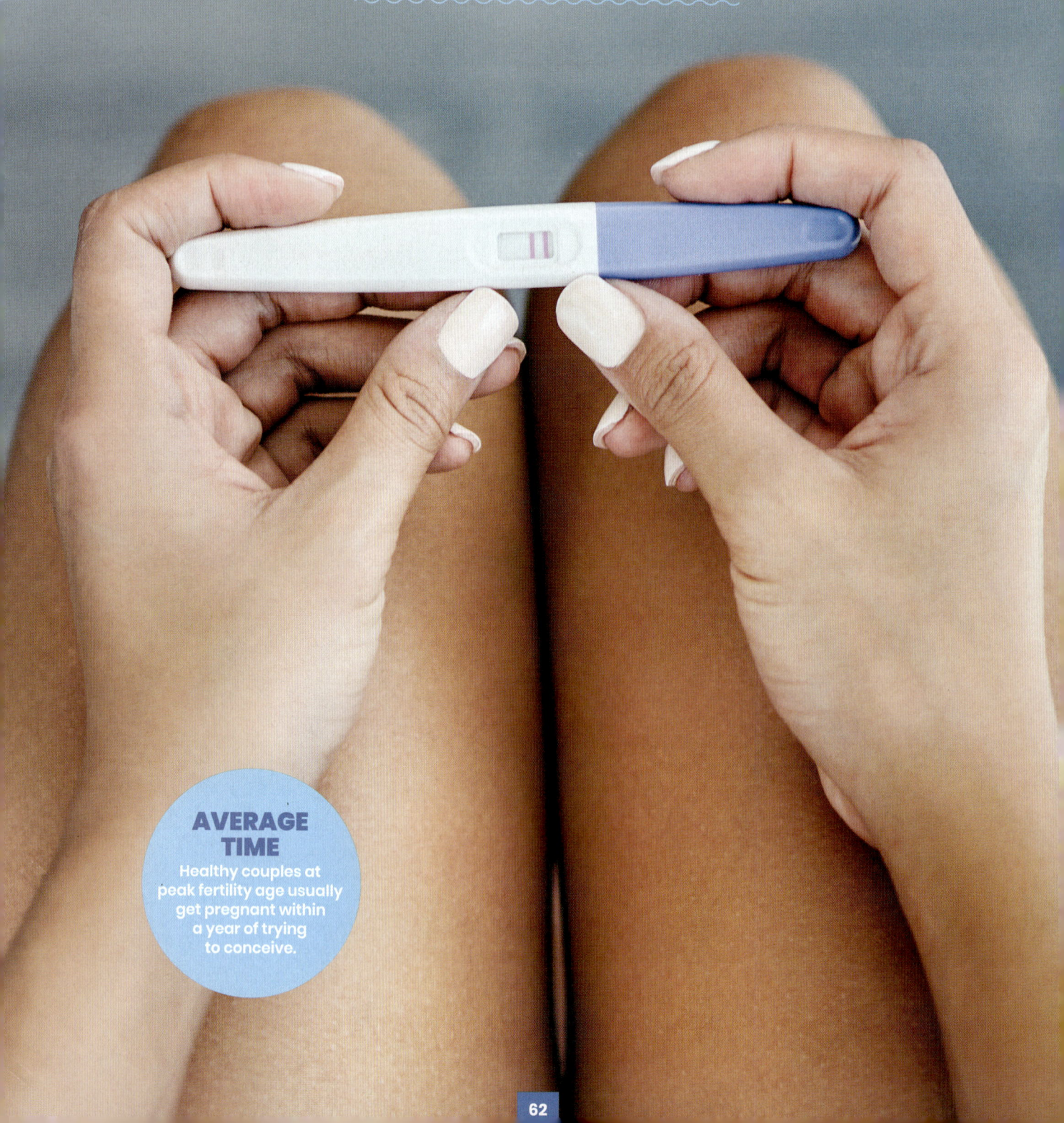

AVERAGE TIME
Healthy couples at peak fertility age usually get pregnant within a year of trying to conceive.

While conceiving a baby is a natural part of human life, that doesn't mean it's easy. There are so many factors that influence our ability to conceive, and even if everything is in our favour, it doesn't mean it will happen overnight. If you are ovulating regularly, are leading a relatively healthy lifestyle, have no underlying conditions and are under 40, then your fertility should be optimum. But it's not always so black and white.

BACK TO BASICS

First, a reminder of how conception works. Following the ovulation phase of your menstrual cycle, a mature egg makes its way down the fallopian tubes towards your uterus. The egg needs to be fertilised within a day of it being released, as it only has a limited time of being viable.

In men, sperm is produced in the testicles; upon ejaculation, millions of sperm cells are released. Sperm is a little more durable than an egg and can hang around in the body for up to three to five days, so if you've had unprotected sex just before, during or just after ovulation, there is the possibility of conception. The sperm enters the vagina and makes its way up to meet the egg in the fallopian tube. Of all the millions of sperm cells, just one will break through the egg's outer cells and fertilise it – but often no sperm cells break through at all and the egg isn't fertilised and is dissolved.

If the egg is successfully fertilised, it becomes known as a zygote, continuing its journey towards the uterus. It now begins the process of cell division, into two cells, then four and so on. It takes about a week until the zygote arrives at the uterus, by which point it is made up of around 100 cells and is now called a blastocyst. This is what implants into the lining of the uterus to continue with pregnancy, however sometimes a fertilised egg doesn't implant and will instead be passed out of the body during menstruation as usual. It's unlikely you would ever know that this has happened.

If implantation is successful, the cells continue to divide and develop, with some cells forming the early stages of a baby and others forming the placenta. This process also triggers the release of hormones to ensure that the body prepares for pregnancy, and you won't have a normal period.

INCREASE YOUR CHANCES

The most obvious thing that you need to do to increase your chances of a healthy conception is to have unprotected penile-vaginal sex. If you're actively trying to have a baby, then the best time to have sex is in the days around ovulation, including before and after. Some people track their ovulation cycles to get the timing right, but this can become quite stressful and can make some people feel a lot of pressure. Unless you have other factors or underlying conditions, then you don't need to be too precise with tracking your cycle. Think about having sex every two to three days without contraception, and focus on enjoyment rather than procreation. This will help your body to be more at ease, which can help with conception.

If you are actively trying for a baby, then you are advised to start taking a folic acid supplement – ideally three months before you start trying. You will then continue to take this for the first 12 weeks of a successful pregnancy. Folic acid is important for ▶

CONCEIVING MULTIPLES

While rare, it is possible to conceive two or more babies at the same time

Multiple births – that is, when more than one baby is born to a woman at a time – are relatively uncommon. Only about 1 in 65 natural births are multiple births.[1] The chance of having identical twins is about 1 in every 250 pregnancies; higher numbers of multiples is even more rare, rising to 1 in every 10,000 births for triplets. There are two different types of twins, which are determined by the way they're conceived. Identical twins are formed when a single fertilised egg splits in two. These are known as monozygotic twins, because both babies come from one identical embryo and they share all their DNA, though they may have differences due to non-genetic factors. Non-identical twins are called dizygotic – they are created when two different eggs are produced at the same time and both are fertilised. Non-identical twins have different sets of DNA, the same as any other set of siblings. If there are triplets, they may all be developed from separate eggs, be from one embryo split three ways, or even a combination where two of the babies are identical and the third baby is non-identical.

Understanding Conception

IN VITRO
FERTILISATION

IVF can be used in some cases to help people who have problems trying to, or are unable to, conceive naturally

IVF is a form of fertility treatment where fertilisation takes place outside the human body. An egg is harvested from a woman's ovaries and fertilised by a sperm in a laboratory. The fertilised egg (embryo) is then returned to a woman's womb to grow and develop as normal. There are many reasons why a person may need to use IVF to conceive a baby. In some cases, the egg is yours and the sperm belongs to your partner, but it is also possible to use donated eggs or sperm to form the embryo. IVF may also be used in situations of surrogacy, where the embryo is placed in a surrogate's womb. If you're undergoing IVF, your natural menstrual cycle will be controlled through medication and the ovaries stimulated to produce multiple eggs (rather than just one). When the eggs are mature, they are removed and fertilised, before one to two embryos are returned to the womb. Success rates are around 32% for women under 35, and it's rarely performed in women over 42 as the success rates are so low.

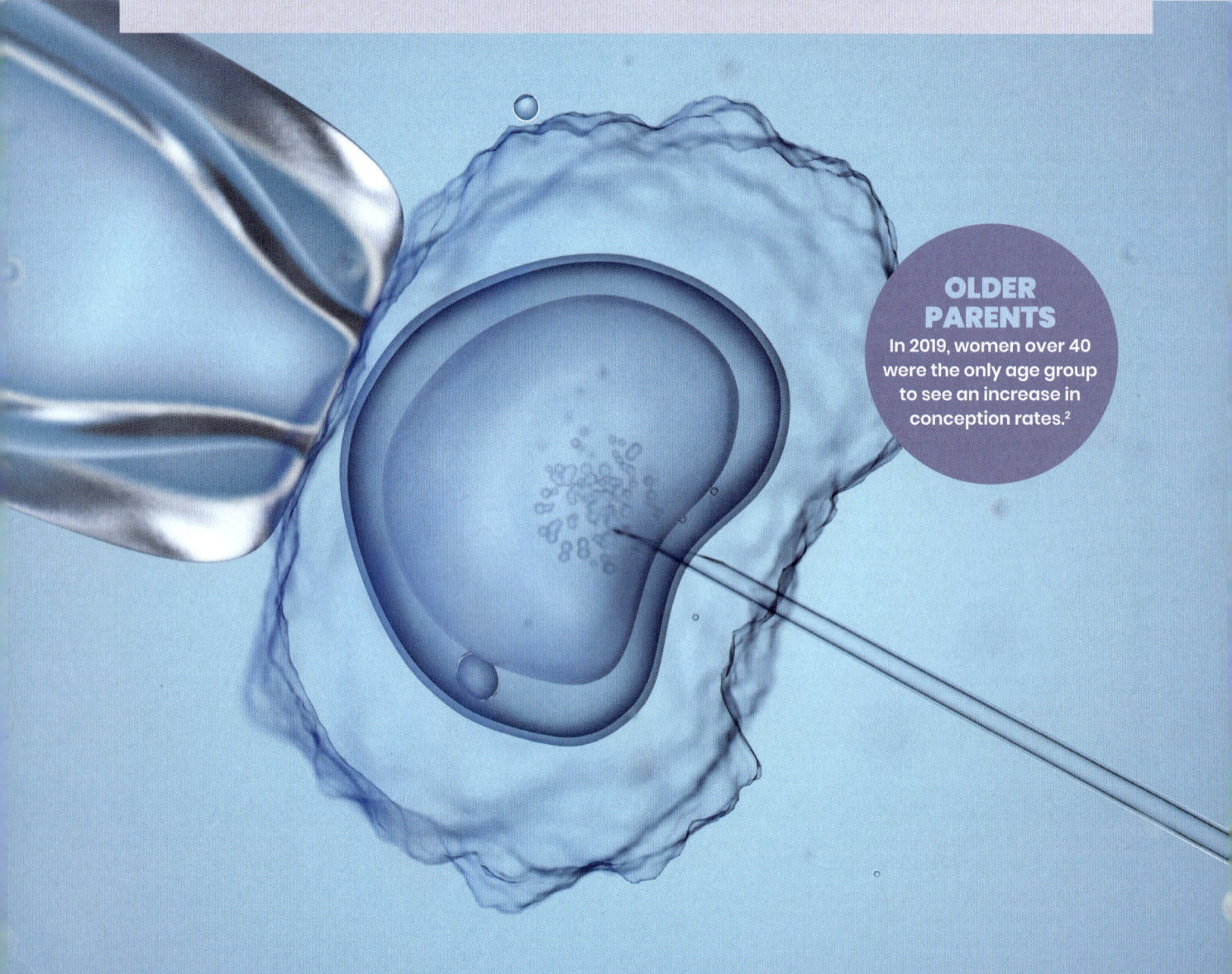

OLDER PARENTS
In 2019, women over 40 were the only age group to see an increase in conception rates.[2]

a baby to develop a healthy brain and spine by helping the body to produce red blood cells. Folic acid is also available naturally in some foods, including broccoli, leafy green vegetables, some beans and peas, fortified cereal or bread, and eggs.

To help increase your chances of conception, you should try to focus on positive lifestyle changes – such as eating a healthy, balanced diet, limiting caffeine and alcohol, exercising regularly and getting plenty of sleep.

> "YOU SHOULD TRY TO FOCUS ON POSITIVE LIFESTYLE CHANGES"

IMPACTS ON CONCEPTION

There are factors that can have a negative impact on your ability to conceive. Your age is the biggest factor, as we know that our fertility declines with every year. That doesn't mean it's impossible to have a baby in later life, just that it might take longer or that you will need some medical help.

We can't change our age, but there are other things we can do that may influence our chances of conception. For example, if you're trying for a baby and you smoke, you should stop. Smoking can harm the delicate lining of the womb and reduce the quantity and quality of your eggs. This is also true of second-hand smoke. Additionally, if a man smokes it can damage the sperm cells and reduce the sperm's mobility. Alcohol consumption is another modifiable factor towards successful conception, as it can disrupt your hormones – as well as damage the quality of your eggs if it is being consumed in excessive quantities.

Your weight can affect your chance of getting pregnant. Being overweight or underweight can reduce your chances of conceiving naturally, as it can impact on your menstrual cycle. Women with a BMI of 30 or more (which is classified as obese), can take longer to get pregnant but also be at a higher risk of complications in pregnancy, including an increased risk of miscarriage. It also makes any fertility treatment less likely to succeed.

If you have an underlying health condition like a hormonal imbalance, an ovarian disorder like PCOS or fibroids, or even a mental health condition, these can all make it harder to conceive, and you will need to speak to your doctor for advice.

WHEN TO SEE A DOCTOR

If you've been trying to conceive for a while, you might be worried that there's a problem. First, it's important to remember that it can take time and that you may need to be patient. Even if everything is alright, you may not conceive straight away. The usual advice is to actively try for a year before seeking medical advice, as it can naturally take that long to get pregnant. Remember, you only have, on average, 12-13 opportunities to get pregnant in a year due to the menstrual cycle and ovulation, and the conditions and timing have to be just right.

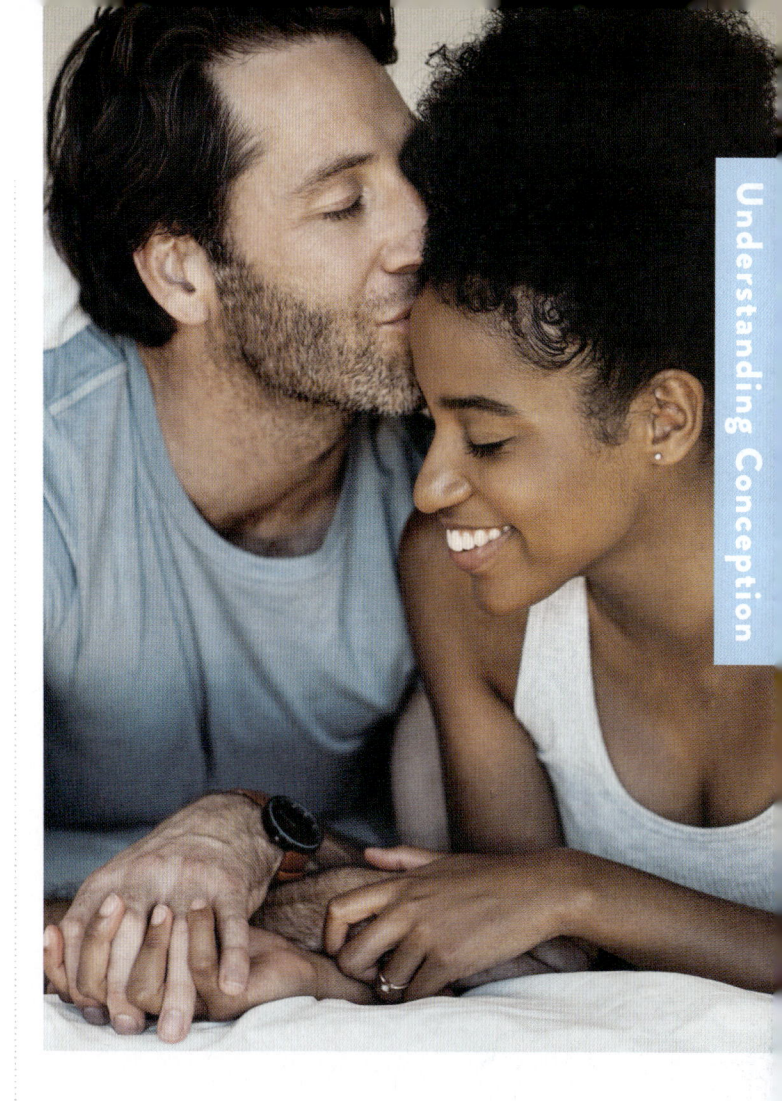

If you go past the year mark, it's worth speaking to your doctor. They can run some tests to see if there are any underlying issues you don't know about. This can include checking both the man and the woman's reproductive capabilities, as well as ruling out medical conditions. If you're over 35, a doctor can give some advice on conception, as it can start to get a little harder from this point.

Some people should get advice from a doctor before trying to conceive. This is true if you have a long-term condition, like diabetes, which might mean you need extra monitoring in pregnancy, or if there is a chance of passing on a condition like sickle cell disease. Some medicines can impact your chances of getting pregnant or could be damaging to an embryo, so again you will need to speak to your doctor before trying for a baby.

If you do conceive, then you're about to start a completely new journey into pregnancy and beyond. This will impact on your physical and mental health, as well as creating huge changes in your body.

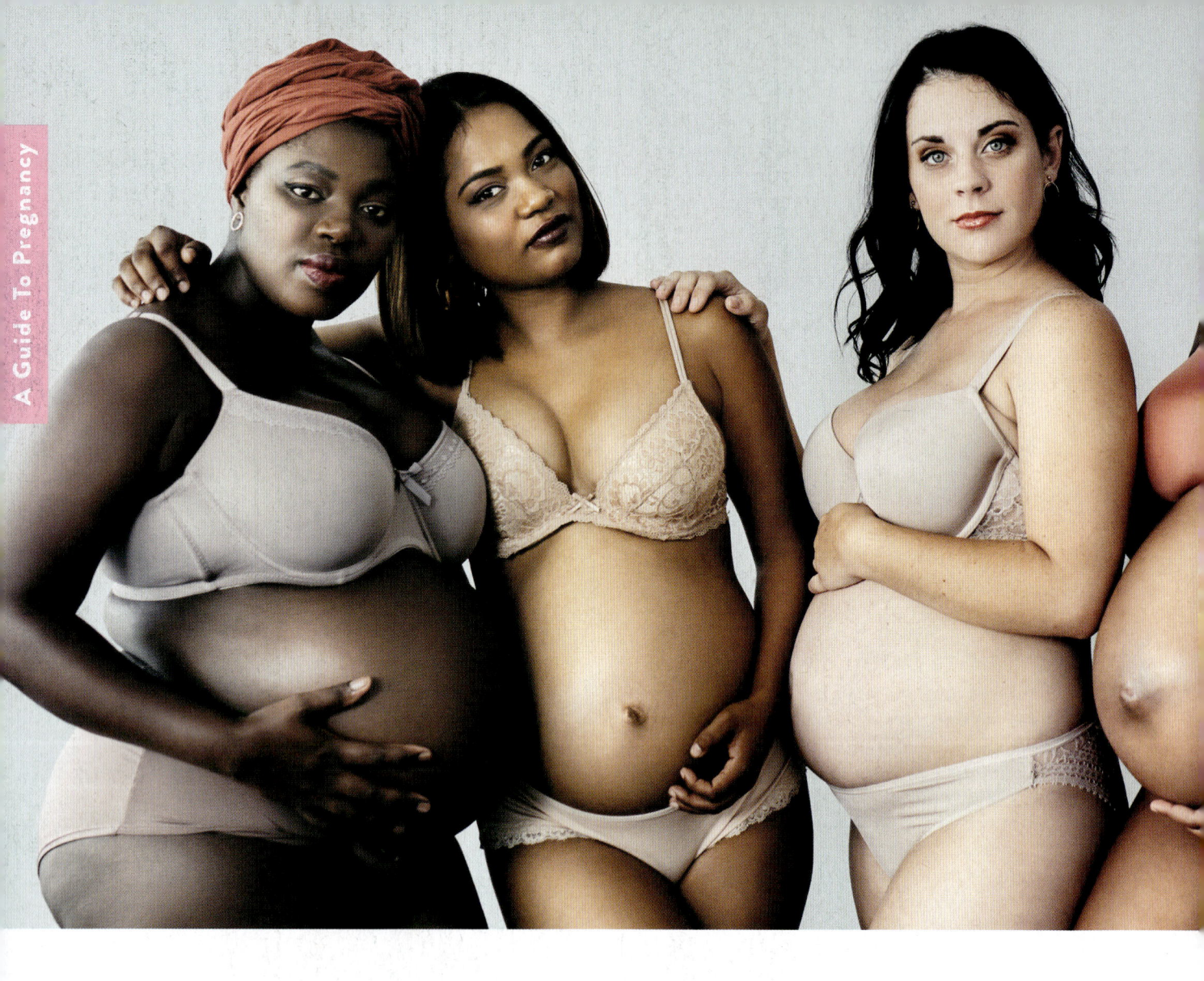

A GUIDE TO PREGNANCY

Here is a quick overview of what you need to know about growing a baby

When you first conceive, you won't know about it for a little while. The body still has some work to do to get ready for the pregnancy, but it won't be too long until you begin to notice some of the early signs. This marks the start of a process that lasts for around nine months, during which time your body will undergo huge changes to grow a baby and ultimately prepare for childbirth.

EARLY PREGNANCY

For many people, the first indication that you are pregnant is when you miss a period. This is easier to determine if you are normally quite regular; if your cycle is generally irregular then it can be more difficult to determine when you've missed a period. Some women do have a light bleed, similar to a period, even though they're pregnant. This can sometimes happen after implantation, and the

JOIN GROUPS
Being part of a pregnancy group can help you feel more supported and connected.

BABY LOSS

Sometimes pregnancy doesn't develop in the way that it should

Sadly, sometimes a pregnancy goes wrong and the baby is not viable. We don't always know why this occurs. More often than not, it's just something that happens and there's nothing that can be done to prevent it. Most commonly, it's due to chromosomal abnormalities that impact proper development. Some women have what's known as an ectopic pregnancy, which is when the fertilised egg implants into the fallopian tube rather than the womb. Sadly, this is not a viable pregnancy and would seriously endanger the health of the mother to continue. Most incidents of baby loss are early miscarriages, which is when the loss happens before 12 weeks. It's estimated that this happens to between 10-20% of pregnancies.[1] Late miscarriage is when the loss happens after 12 weeks and before 24 weeks, which is estimated to affect 3-4% of pregnancies. For every week you are pregnant, the risk of a loss lowers. If the baby dies beyond 24 weeks, this is known as stillbirth and can obviously be incredibly traumatic. In England, this happens in around 1 in 250 births and there is support available for these sad circumstances.

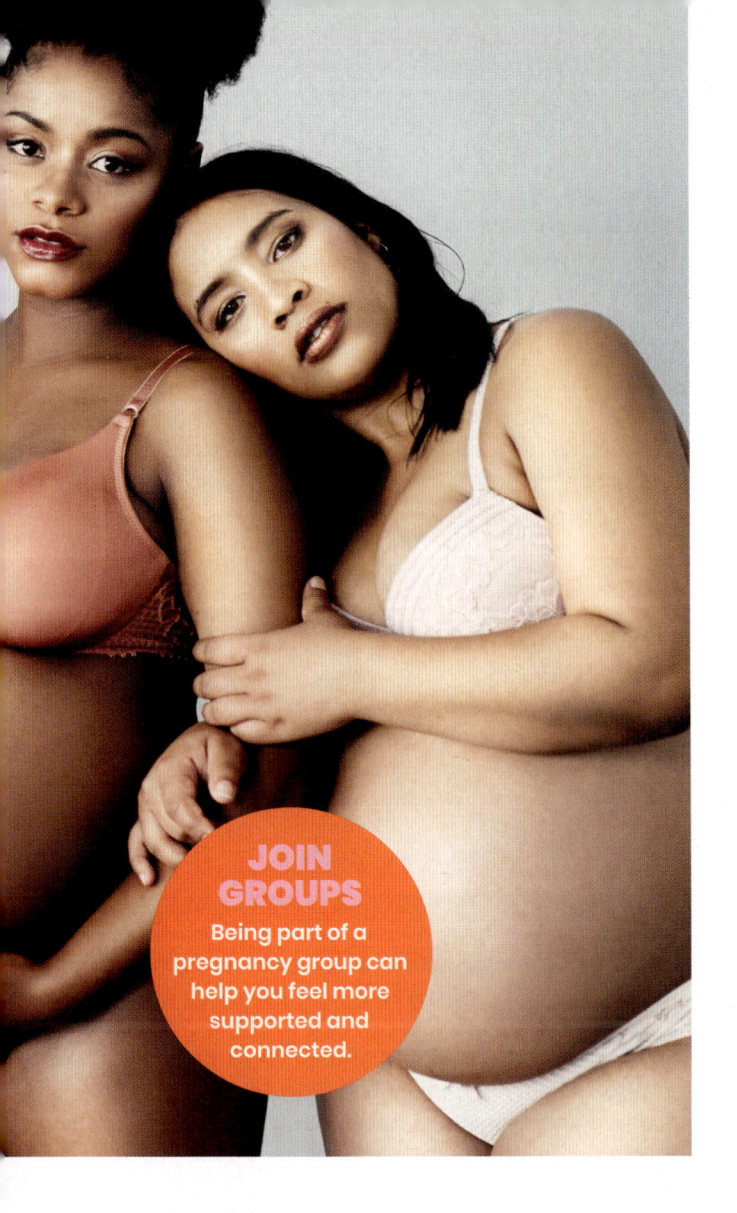

> **"HOME TESTING KITS ARE FAIRLY RELIABLE – FALSE POSITIVES ARE RARE"**

blood loss is usually light in comparison to a normal period.

It's around this time of a missed period that many women take a pregnancy test. Pregnancy tests can be performed quickly and easily at home or at your doctor's surgery. Home testing kits are fairly reliable. The tests check your hCG levels, which rise rapidly in early pregnancy. Most tests involve urinating on a plastic test stick and waiting a small amount of time before reading the result. A positive result is usually accurate – false positives on home tests, while possible, are rare. If you test too soon, however, you may get a negative result even if you are pregnant. If there is a chance you are pregnant, you may wish to repeat the test again a week later. Once you get a positive result, you would usually make an appointment to see your doctor and start the process of getting set up for prenatal care.

From about four to six weeks of pregnancy, you may start to notice some changes. Many women find that their first symptom is sore or tender breasts. Your breasts may also feel swollen or sensitive, or change in appearance, including a darkening of the nipple. You may start to feel more tired than usual, which can be due to the hormonal changes that are happening in your body.

Some women also start to feel sick, or actually be sick, commonly called morning sickness (though it doesn't only happen in the morning). In the early days of pregnancy, you may also need to urinate more often than usual or you may become more constipated. You may also find that you start to ▶

A Guide To Pregnancy

▶ have cravings for different foods, or find the smell or taste of things unappealing.

Once you've had a positive pregnancy test, you can calculate your rough due date. There are calculators available online, which use the first date of your last period and your typical cycle length. You will get an updated due date once you've had your first scan. The length of pregnancy can vary, so although you might have a due date, that doesn't determine when your baby will actually arrive.

FIRST TRIMESTER

In the first trimester, which comprises the first 12 weeks of pregnancy, those early symptoms can carry on. It's not uncommon to feel fatigued, need to pee a lot, have heavy and swollen breasts, and experience some morning sickness. The initial rush of hormones can have a big impact on your physical and mental state.

Many women find the first trimester an emotional time. This is normal – your body is changing, but you also start to come to terms with the fact that you're growing a baby and what that means for your life. At this point, the foetus is tiny. By six weeks, it is about the size of a pea; by 10 weeks a strawberry; and by the end of the first trimester, a plum. So, while you might be feeling very pregnant, it's unlikely that anyone else would notice unless you choose to tell them. Your stomach may get a little more rounded, but you probably won't have a noticeable baby bump quite yet – you may show sooner in future pregnancies.

> **"YOU MIGHT FIND YOU START TO FEEL A BIT BETTER AS YOU MOVE INTO THE SECOND TRIMESTER"**

At around 12 weeks you will have an ultrasound scan, which is sometimes called a 'dating' scan. This is an important scan that checks how the baby is developing and if there are any underlying issues. Various measurements are taken on-screen to help determine your baby's due date.

Many women choose not to tell anyone about their pregnancy until after this scan. There is a higher risk of things going wrong in the early stages of pregnancy, which is why it's not uncommon to keep the news within a close circle until the 12-week scan has been performed. There is no right time to tell anyone about the pregnancy if you don't want to – you're under no obligation. In the UK, you need to tell your employer that you're pregnant at least

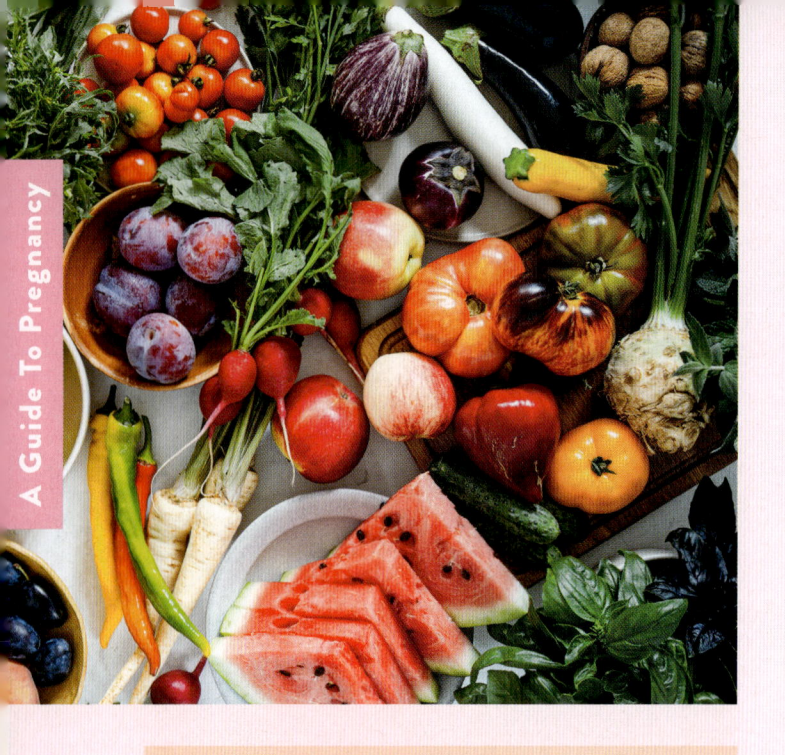

NUTRITION TIPS FOR PREGNANCY

Eating well can help your baby's development as well as boost your own health

When you're pregnant, it's important to stay healthy and make sure that you're getting enough nutritious foods to ensure that you stay strong and healthy. There isn't a specific pregnancy diet; just try to eat a healthy, balanced range of foods, high in fruits and vitamins, wholegrains, lean protein, some dairy and healthy fats. Try to limit intake of ultraprocessed foods high in sugar and fat. There is a myth that you have to 'eat for two' when pregnant, but you don't need to. You may need to eat slightly more than usual to keep your energy up, but this is an extra snack or two, or slightly larger meal portions, rather than doubling up! There are some foods you need to avoid in pregnancy due to the risk of infection – such as certain cheeses, paté, some fish and raw eggs – but your prenatal team should give you a list. You also need to drink plenty of water and limit caffeine.

15 weeks before the due date, but if you're struggling with symptoms, you may need to tell them earlier so that any reasonable adjustments can be made. You may also need to arrange time off for medical appointments. This process will be different depending on where you're based.

There are various professionals who may be involved in your care during your pregnancy. This depends on whether you are using private or state services, what you're covered for by insurance, and where in the world you are. It's important that you attend all prenatal checks, as these are designed to keep an eye on your baby's health as well as your own.

SECOND TRIMESTER

You might find that you start to feel a bit better as you move into the second trimester. Some of this is because the risk of the pregnancy going wrong drops, which can help with any anxiety. Many women find this the most enjoyable trimester of the whole pregnancy, going from 13 weeks through to 28 weeks.

Early pregnancy symptoms can start to taper off, with morning sickness coming to an end for many women and energy levels rising. Everyone is different, though, so it's not unusual to still have some symptoms. During this trimester, your body will change more obviously, and by the end of these months you will have a visible bump.

It's during this trimester that you have more important tests. This may include blood tests and additional scans, but if your pregnancy is progressing as expected, then the next big routine scan is the 20-week anomaly scan. By 20 weeks, the baby is about the size of a banana and all the major organs are developing. The anomaly scan checks for a range of different conditions that can impact on development, such as spina bifida, cleft lip and any cardiac abnormalities, for example. Other things are checked too, such as the blood flow into your uterus, your placenta function and the length of the baby from heel to toe.

During the second trimester you should also start to feel the baby moving for the first time. Normally this occurs any time from around 16 weeks, but it can take longer in first-time pregnancies. The first ▶

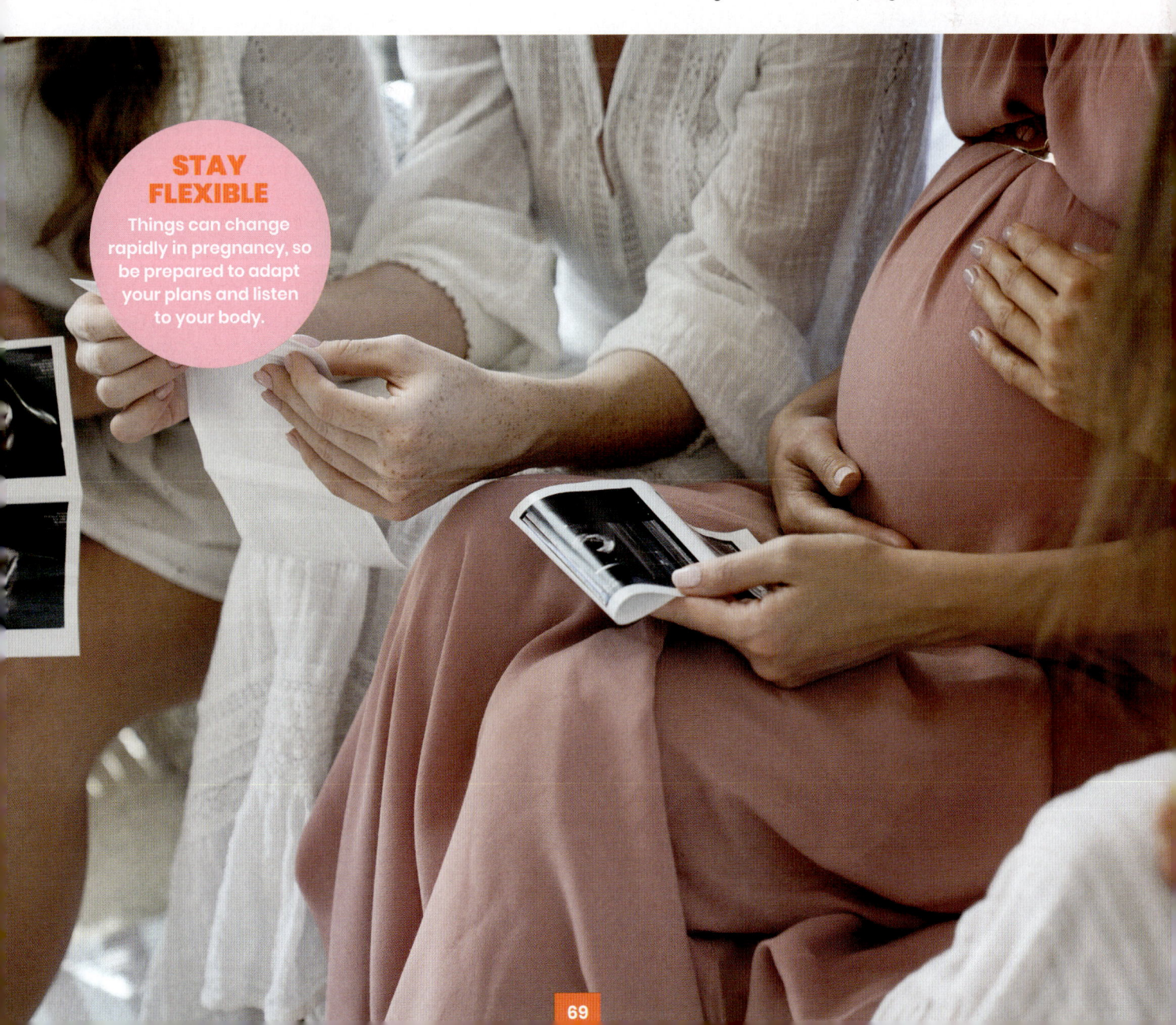

A Guide To Pregnancy

STAY FLEXIBLE
Things can change rapidly in pregnancy, so be prepared to adapt your plans and listen to your body.

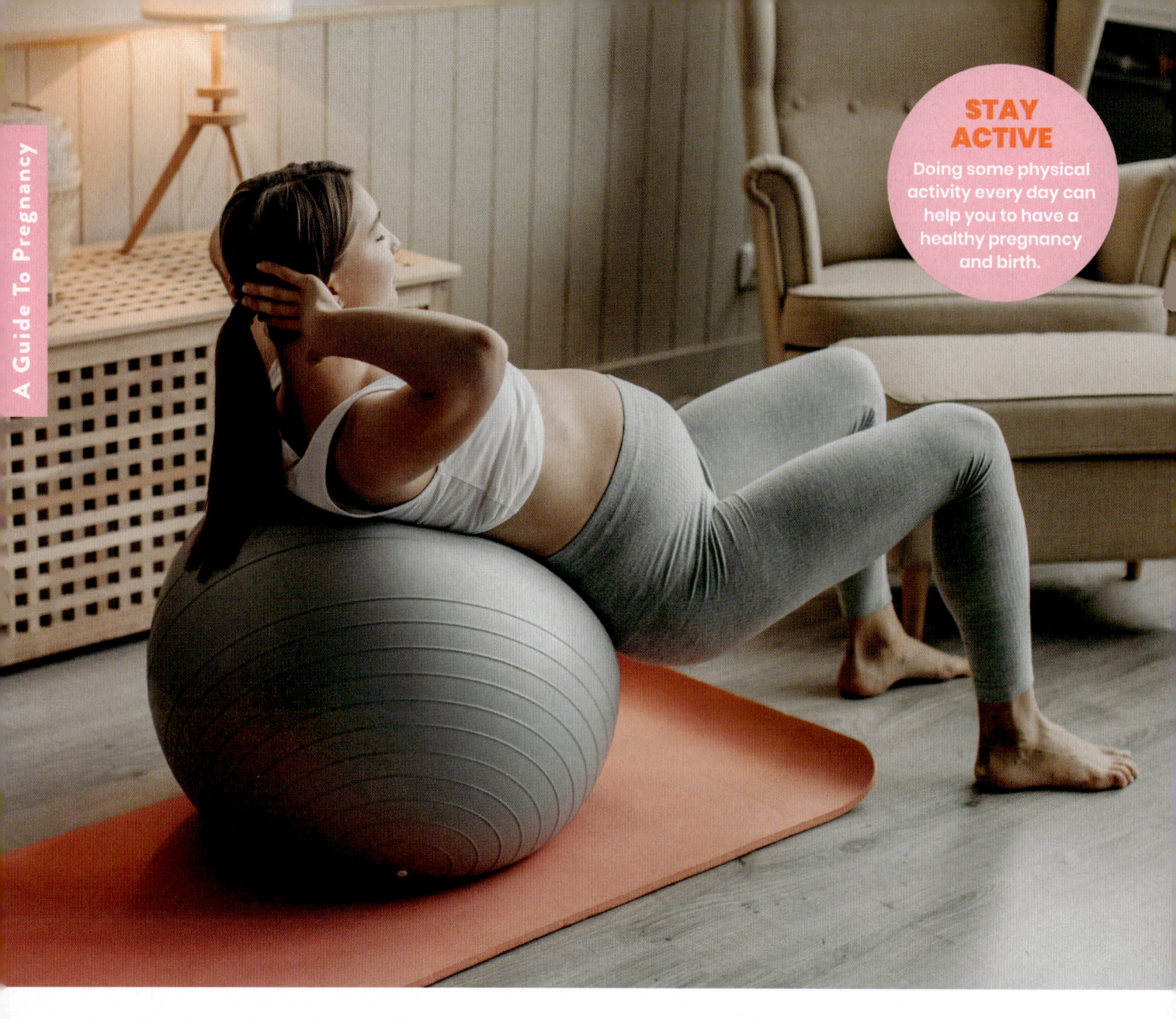

STAY ACTIVE
Doing some physical activity every day can help you to have a healthy pregnancy and birth.

▸ movements are not the strong kicks you may feel later on; they're more subtle, often described as a fluttering sensation, called 'quickening'.

THIRD TRIMESTER

The final stage of pregnancy, which lasts from 29 weeks until the baby is born, is when your body might start to tell you to slow down. Your bump will grow a lot more and that can become very tiring. It can affect your back and legs, due to the front-loaded weight that you're carrying around. You may start to find some daily activities more difficult, but it's important to stay active as this can help with both your health and your baby's health, as well as help prepare for the stamina and strength needed for labour and post-partum recovery.

You will likely see your prenatal team more often as you get nearer to the end of your pregnancy. The most important things that they're looking for are any underlying issues that could affect the birth, as well as the position of the baby. At some point before labour, your baby should get into the right position to be born, which is head down and facing your back. This is called the occiput-anterior (OA) position and is the most common position for a baby to move into because it makes it easier to give birth naturally. However, if your baby is not in this position, this will be monitored. Other positions can make labour last longer and be more difficult, and also raise the chance of needing intervention to help with the birth.

At some point, again towards the end of your pregnancy, the baby's head will drop down into your pelvis and engage. This can feel uncomfortable, but it is a sign that your baby is almost ready to be born.

PREGNANCY COMPLICATIONS

With all pregnancies, there is a small risk of complications. Some are more serious than others,

"THE FINAL STAGE OF PREGNANCY IS WHEN YOUR BODY TELLS YOU TO SLOW DOWN"

PREPARING TO GIVE BIRTH

Get ready for the next stage by starting to think about your birth plan

In the third trimester, you will probably start to think more about the actual birth and what that will be like. You may want to make a birth plan, which is an outline of your wishes for the birth. This might include where you want to give birth, what pain relief you want, whether you want a water birth or not, and what you want to happen after the birth. While it's a good idea to have an idea of what you want and the opportunity to discuss it with your prenatal team, you need to be flexible. Anything can happen in labour – you may change your mind and want different pain relief, or you might be advised that part of your plan is no longer possible. The priority is that both you and your baby are healthy, so stay open-minded and adaptable. At the end of the day, even if the birth doesn't go to plan, having a strong and healthy baby is the most important thing.

but it's important to attend all prenatal checks to ensure that any issues are picked up as soon as possible so that treatment can begin quickly.

Most morning sickness passes over time, but if you're being sick a lot and struggling to keep food down, then you may have a condition called hyperemesis gravidarum (HG), which is a serious condition and requires medical treatment. Having HG can make it more difficult to ensure you're getting enough nutrients in for both your body and your baby's development.

Your blood pressure will be monitored throughout the pregnancy, as having high blood pressure (hypertension) can be a sign that your body is struggling. It can also be a sign of pre-eclampsia, which is when a problem with your placenta causes a rise in blood pressure that can impact on your organs and brain. It can be dangerous for both you and your baby, so your prenatal team will be checking for early warning signs. It is more common if you have a family history of pre-eclampsia in pregnancies and if you already have hypertension before getting pregnant.

Another risk, although rare, is developing deep vein thrombosis (DVT). This is when a blood clot forms in a vein, usually in the leg. It can break off and block the blood vessels in the lungs (called a pulmonary embolism). It's a serious condition that has to be treated immediately. Your risk factor in pregnancy is higher than someone of the same age who is not pregnant, but it's still a tiny risk. Some things make the risk higher, such as being over 35, being obese, carrying multiple babies or having a family history of blood clots.

It's important not to worry too much about these kinds of complications, as they are uncommon. Most women will have healthy pregnancies, but you are also being well monitored the whole time. And as you get to the end of the pregnancy, your thoughts will likely start to turn to the birth and everything that's yet to come.

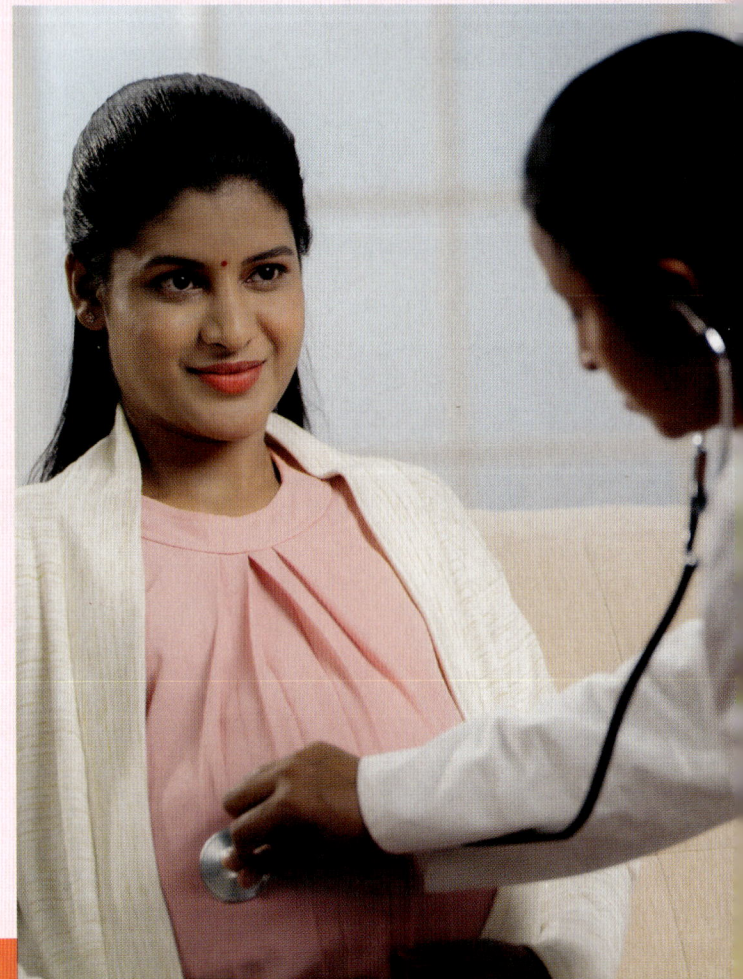

LABOUR & BIRTH

Coming to the end of pregnancy can feel like a relief, but labour and birth take a toll on the body

Somewhere around 280 days (40 weeks) from the start of your last period, your body will start showing signs of labour, the point at which your baby is ready to be born. That's just an average; the majority of babies are born between 37 and 42 weeks. A baby is considered to be 'full term' at 37 weeks, which means that they have fully developed everything they need to survive outside the womb. Babies born before 37 weeks are pre-term, and depending on how early they are born, they may need specialist care (see the box on page 74).

SIGNS OF LABOUR

As you approach the end of your pregnancy, you should notice the signs of labour (unless you have a planned procedure to deliver the baby earlier). The most common and obvious sign of labour is when contractions begin. Contractions are when the muscles in your uterus tighten and then relax, to prepare your body for childbirth and moving a baby through your vaginal canal. These contractions begin slowly and are irregular; they may feel similar to cramps during a menstrual period. As the labour progresses, they will get deeper, more intense and closer together. They can be very painful, which is why there are various forms of pain relief available to labouring women. Some types of pain relief might not be suitable at the start or not right for your situation, but your prenatal team will help you with your options, depending on how you're coping.

> **"THE MAJORITY OF BABIES ARE BORN BETWEEN 37 WEEKS, WHICH IS FULL-TERM, AND 42 WEEKS"**

AFTER THE BIRTH

What happens in the hours after a baby is born

It's easy to get wrapped up in the labour and birth phase of pregnancy without giving much thought to what comes next. Where possible, a newborn baby will be placed on your skin straight after birth, ideally even before the umbilical cord has been cut. This is called skin-to-skin contact. It helps with bonding between mother and baby, and can also help with establishing a first breastfeed once the baby is ready and if the mother chooses to do so. The baby will be towelled down to remove any blood or other substances from their skin, and wrapped up to keep them warm. In some cases, the newborn will need to be checked over by the medical team present to ensure everything is as it should be. The baby will also be weighed and measured. Babies are often given a vitamin K injection straight away (though you can opt out), which helps to prevent a rare bleeding disorder in newborns. At the same time, you will be looked after, with repairs to any tears that have happened during the birth and the team ensuring you're comfortable.

WORLDWIDE BIRTHRATE

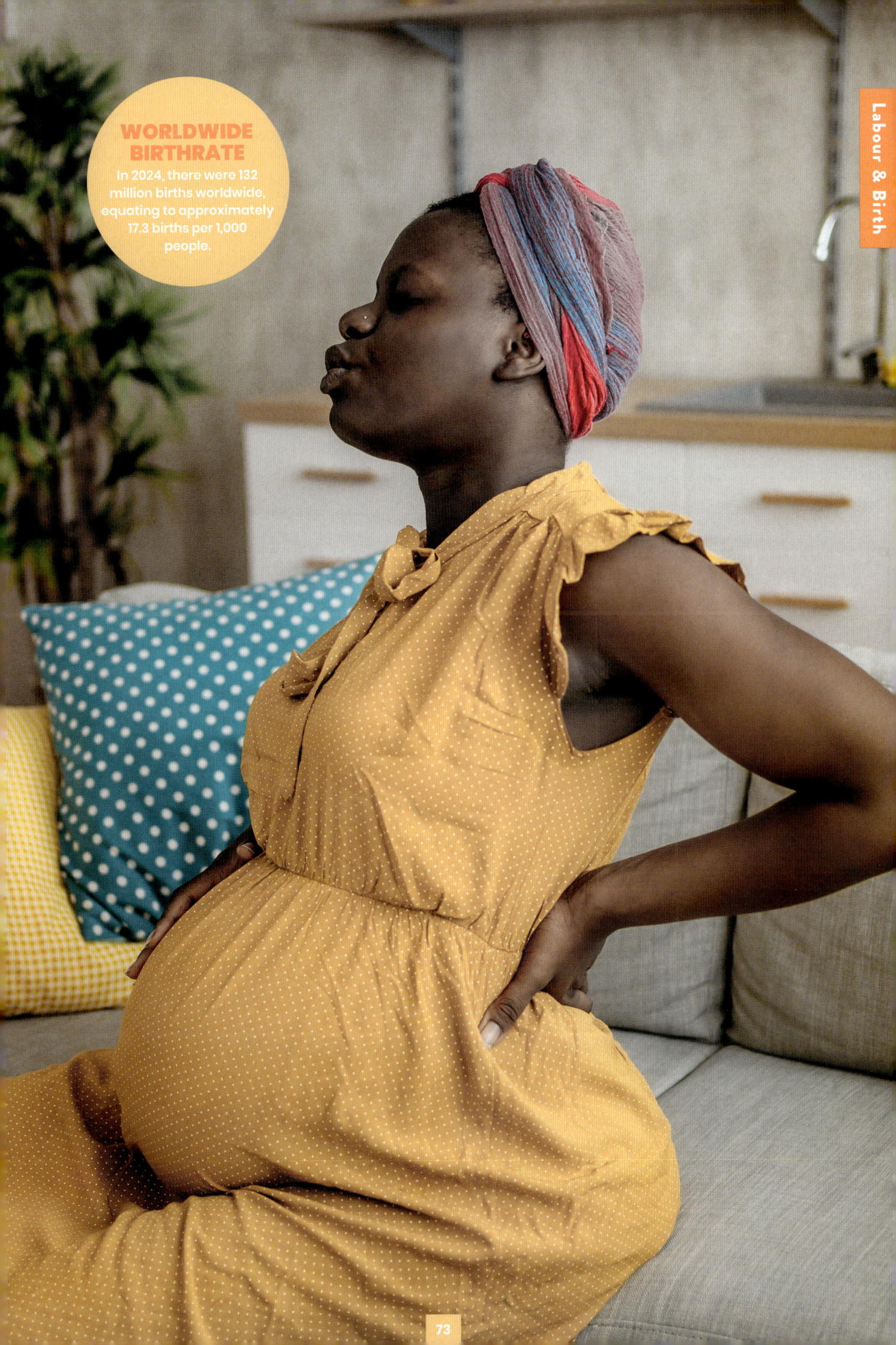

In 2024, there were 132 million births worldwide, equating to approximately 17.3 births per 1,000 people.

Labour & Birth

PRE-TERM BIRTH

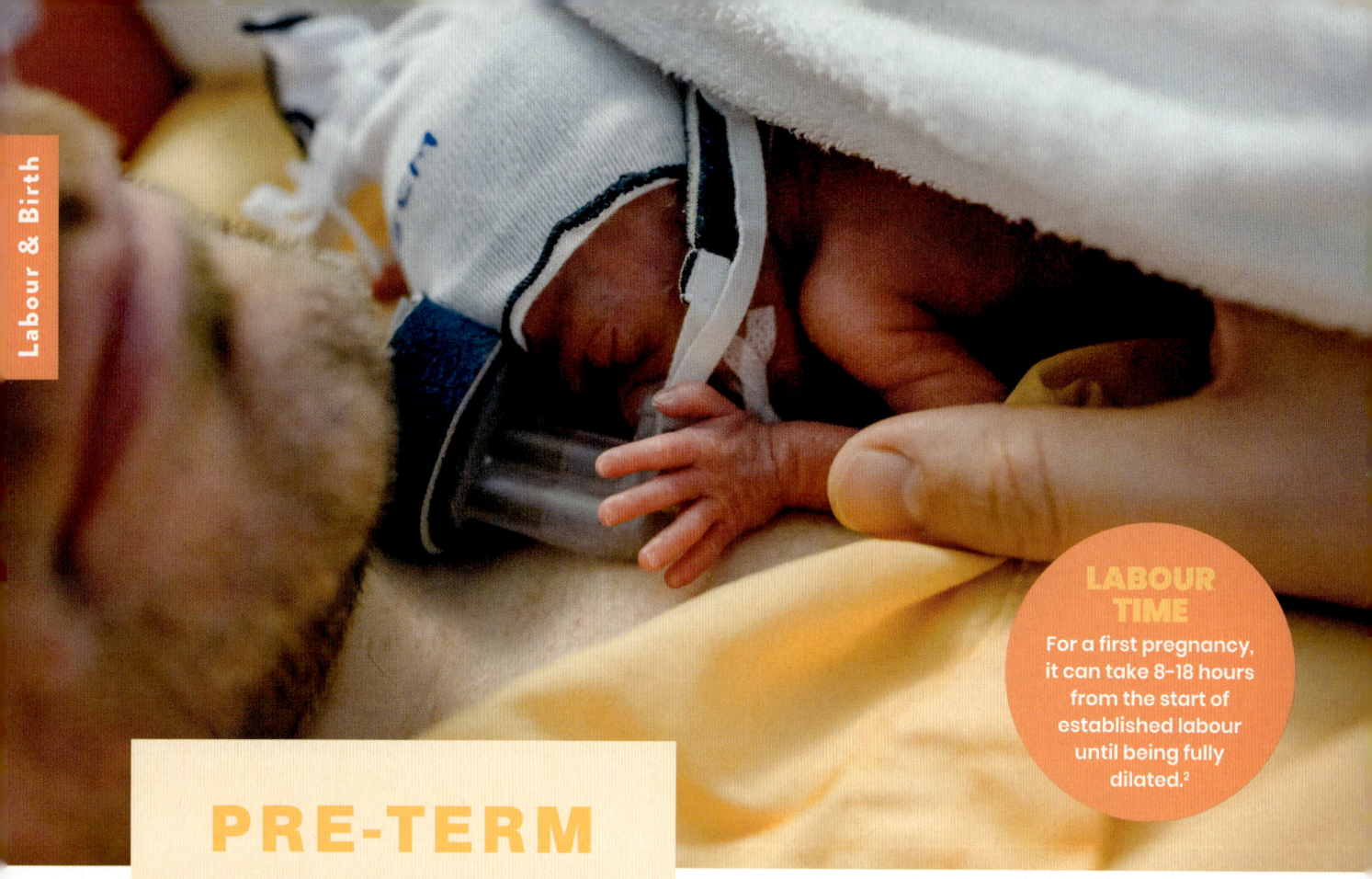

Around 8 in 100 babies are born before 37 weeks[1]

Pre-term babies are at higher risk of post-birth complications. Going into early labour can happen for a number of different reasons. Sometimes a baby needs to be born earlier because continuing with the pregnancy could put the mother's or the baby's health in danger. Other times, labour starts early by itself and is more common in multiple pregnancies. If signs of labour do start early, and there are no underlying health reasons that mean the birth needs to take place, there are medical treatments that can slow down or stop the labour to give the baby more time to develop, as well as medicine for the baby to help strengthen their lungs. It is possible for babies to survive from 24 weeks, but they will need a lot of support in a neonatal unit and may face developmental issues. Babies born between 32 and 37 weeks are considered moderate to late premature and have a lower risk of serious complications; over 80% of babies born pre-term fall in this category.

LABOUR TIME
For a first pregnancy, it can take 8-18 hours from the start of established labour until being fully dilated.[2]

▸ Another sign of labour is something that not all women notice or have. There is a 'plug' of mucus around the cervix, which helps to protect the uterus from infection. This can be loosened out of place during labour, passing out through the vagina – this is sometimes called a 'show'. Other symptoms include intense backache and needing, or feeling the urge, to go to the toilet as the baby presses against your bowel and bladder. You may also notice your waters breaking, which is when the amniotic sac surrounding your baby in the womb ruptures and the fluid leaks out. This usually happens in the first stage of labour, but if your waters break and contractions haven't started, you may need to be monitored as it increases the risk of infection.

STAGES OF LABOUR

Labour is broken down into different stages. There is a pre-labour phase, sometimes called the latent stage, which is when the cervix starts to dilate (open up to allow the baby to pass through) and some irregular, early contractions begin. During this time, you should focus on fuelling your body for the impending birth, drinking water and resting or sleeping if you can.

The first stage of labour is called established labour, which is determined by strong and regular contractions, as well as a dilation of the cervix of around 4cm. This is usually when you would call your birthing unit if you're still at home to get advice. You don't have to go into the hospital or birthing unit (if that's where you're having the baby) straight away, as this stage can take a long time to progress and you may be more comfortable at home. This stage lasts from the start of established labour until your cervix is fully dilated, which is around 10cm. Many women find it hard to rest during this phase and it's not uncommon to want to move around, walking or bouncing on a pregnancy ball.

> **"YOUR BABY MAY NEED A LITTLE EXTRA HELP TO COME OUT"**

Every labour is different; you may be monitored from the very beginning or it can be very hands off until you're ready to give birth. Problems can arise during labour, so your prenatal team should have given you things to watch out for or tell them about.

Once your cervix is fully dilated, you may start to feel an urge to push. The baby will move further into the birth canal. In this stage of labour, you will need to push gently when you have a contraction. With each push, your baby moves further down the canal towards the entrance of your vagina. Breathing exercises can help you to stay calm and focus on the pushing. This stage should take no more than three hours (first baby) or two hours (subsequent babies), but it can be much quicker. Once the baby's head is visible ('crowning'), you'll be advised to slow down and stop pushing so that your baby can be born slowly, which can help to prevent tears. After the head is out, the baby will be born quickly, within a couple of contractions.

There is also a third stage of labour. This is the birth of the placenta, which also comes out through the birth canal and vagina via contractions. It is much easier to pass than the baby, as it is soft and flexible. In some cases, you can wait for this to happen naturally, or you can have what's called 'active management'. This involves being injected with a medicine that makes your womb contract and push out the placenta quickly. This is shown to speed up this phase and reduce the risk of heavy bleeding, but it can make you feel nauseous. This isn't always done immediately, as it's often advised to allow the baby to stay attached to the placenta via the umbilical cord for a few minutes while they adjust. Normally the placenta is delivered within 30 minutes of the baby when using the active management technique.

ASSISTED BIRTH

The above process describes a natural birth with no intervention, but that's not always possible. Sometimes, labour might not be progressing fast enough, which means that medical help may be required to speed things up. Interventions can include breaking your waters manually in order to signal to the body to progress, making your contractions stronger and more regular. If this doesn't work, the next step is to use a type of medicine, called oxytocin or syntocinon, which can make contractions come on more regularly and stronger. In both of these cases, you may be offered additional pain relief, as the change in contractions can be quite sudden. The baby will also need to be monitored to ensure that they're not in any distress during the process.

You may also need an assisted delivery, which is when the baby needs a little extra help to come out. The main methods of assisted vaginal birth include the use of forceps, which are similar to curved tongs, which gently grip the baby's head and help to pull them through the birth canal and out of the vagina. A ventouse, or vacuum cup, can also be used, which uses suction to pull the baby out.

If a vaginal birth is not possible for whatever reason, or there is a problem during labour, you may need a caesarean section (C-section) instead. This is when the baby is delivered via a cut through your stomach and into the womb. Many C-sections are planned procedures when it's determined that this is the safest way to deliver the baby. This could be due to the position of the baby, issues with the placenta, or if you have pre-eclampsia. Planned C-sections will usually be carried out around 39 weeks to limit the chance of you going into natural labour and so that the baby is well developed. A C-section can also be an emergency procedure if a vaginal birth is not progressing or if something goes wrong.

Your body goes through a lot during childbirth and there is a lot of healing to do. Making your postpartum health a priority can help you to recover quicker, which is beneficial for you and your baby.

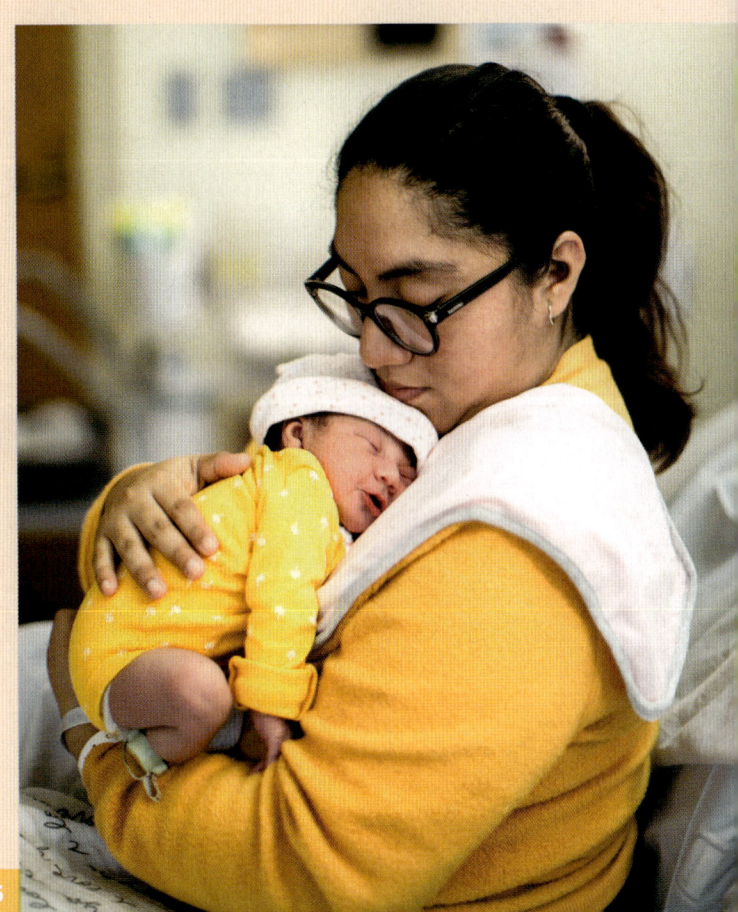

Postpartum Health

POSTNATAL DEPRESSION PREVALENCE
1 in 10 are affected by postnatal depression within a year of giving birth.[1]

POSTPARTUM
HEALTH

What to expect in the days, weeks and months after having a baby

In the days and months following the birth of a baby, your body can feel like it's never going to be the same again. It needs time to heal properly so you can regain your strength and fitness over time. The most important thing is to be kind to yourself and move slowly. You won't be able to pick straight back up where you left off, and how quickly you can get back to your normal activities depends on your general health, how your pregnancy was, how the birth went and how you heal.

POST-BIRTH HEALTH

After giving birth, there is a period of healing. If you had any stitches during childbirth, these may cause a little pain and discomfort. The cuts and tears will heal up, though you will have to be careful about looking after them to prevent infection. Going to the toilet can be uncomfortable too, so it's advised to drink a lot of water so that you're passing diluted urine that won't sting quite as much.

The thought of having a bowel movement after birth can be scary, especially if you are very sore and have a lot of stitches. It's normal to not go straight away: it can be three days or more before you do. You should keep up a healthy diet and drink plenty of water to prevent constipation – which is a possibility due to the increased hormone activity around the birth – but you may need a gentle laxative to help you get things moving, especially if you're avoiding going to the toilet because of a fear it might hurt. Some women find that holding tissue or a maternity pad over the stitches at the same time can help. Another issue that might impact you going to the toilet is that it's quite common to develop haemorrhoids (piles), which can last for a few weeks.

It's also normal to bleed after the birth. This bleed, called lochia, is heavier than a normal period and you will need heavy-duty maternity pads. It's not advised to use a tampon for at least the first six weeks. This bleeding will last for a few weeks, but it will get less heavy until it stops. Women who breastfeed may find that feeding causes the bleeding to be heavier, but if there are large clots then this is something that needs to be checked out.

> **"MANY WOMEN FEEL LOW AND ANXIOUS AT FIRST, WHICH IS A NORMAL FEELING"**

THE EARLY DAYS

The early days after giving birth can be hard both mentally and physically. Many women feel low and anxious at first, which is a normal feeling. You have been through a huge amount, and you are now trying to process that while also meeting the needs of a new person who depends on you. If you still feel low after two weeks, or the periods of ▶

POSTNATAL DEPRESSION

If the baby blues won't go away, you may have postnatal depression

Postnatal depression is a period of low mood that comes on after having a baby, though the symptoms are similar to general depression. Perfectly normal 'baby blues' may last for around two weeks after giving birth, but postnatal depression lasts longer and can occur later on. Symptoms include a feeling of sadness that won't go away, a lack of enjoyment or pleasure in the things you usually enjoy, finding it hard to do normal daily activities, insomnia, intrusive thoughts and having trouble concentrating. Some women hide their symptoms because they worry about whether others will think they can't cope with their new child – but many women have postnatal depression, and it can be treated. It's no reflection on you or your abilities as a parent; it's an illness that needs treatment like any other. Seeking help can prevent it from getting worse and ensure you're accessing the support you need.

Postpartum Health

▶ feeling blue are happening frequently or start later on after the birth, you should speak to someone to get help for possible postnatal depression (see the box on the previous page).

You're also probably not getting enough sleep, which can make you feel emotional. Babies can be very demanding and this can take its toll on your energy levels. It's important to get enough sleep, though, as it will help your body recover in those early days. This means grabbing naps when you can, which can be when your baby sleeps or when you have someone to hold them for you. It isn't easy and sleep will be hard to come by for a while, but anything you can get will help.

Somewhere around six weeks you should get a full postnatal check-up, which makes sure that you're doing okay and that your body is healing. It's normally after this check that you get cleared to start being more active, but not everyone is ready. It's a good idea to move when you can, getting out for gentle walks and doing some stretches. You can start your pelvic floor exercises before your check-up though, as these help to strengthen the muscles in your pelvic organs and help them recover from the trauma of childbirth. Your healthcare team can explain how to do them properly.

With your weakened pelvic floor, you may find that you have less bladder control than you did previously, which can mean you leak urine when you laugh or cough, or on impact. If pelvic floor exercises don't help to tighten up the muscles and prevent leakage, you may need to see a women's health physiotherapist to solve the underlying issue.

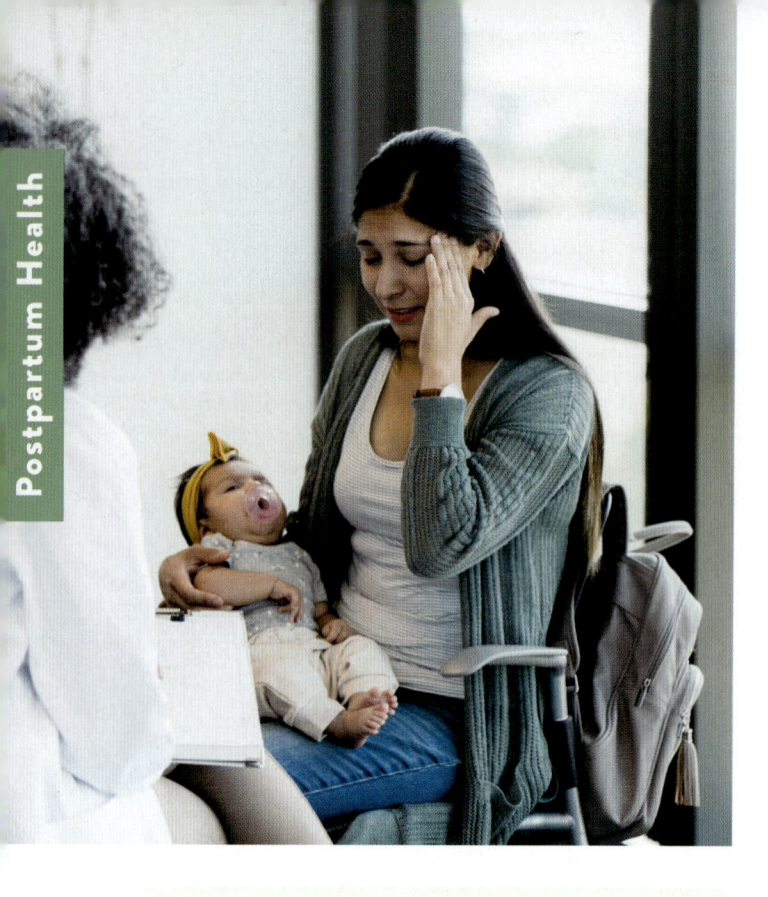

SEX AFTER PREGNANCY

It might not be on your mind for a while, but here's the lowdown

You can start having sex as soon as you feel ready after having baby – there is no timescale. The important thing is that you want to, don't feel pressured to do so and are comfortable enough with your partner to talk about any pain or discomfort you're feeling. Many women don't feel ready for a little while, due to a combination of post-birth bleeding, soreness, stitches and exhaustion. When you are ready, you may need to use extra lubrication to make it more comfortable and take it slowly. If it's especially painful, you may need to give it a little more time, but you can still find other ways to be close to your partner. It might need a little patience, but you can get your usual sex life back on track in time. If you're struggling and it is very sore, you can also get advice from your healthcare team.

> **"IF YOU'RE BREASTFEEDING, YOUR BABY WILL FEED QUITE A LOT IN THE EARLY DAYS"**

BREASTFEEDING AND ITS IMPACT

Your breasts are probably feeling a little sore and tender at this time, too. They will be producing breast milk, starting off with nutrient-rich yellow colostrum. After a few days your breasts will begin producing normal breast milk, which can be uncomfortable at first. If you're breastfeeding, then your baby will feed quite a lot in these early days, and it can feel like you're constantly feeding. It will take a few weeks, but eventually you might settle into a pattern.

While you're producing milk, you may also find that you leak sometimes. You can get breast pads that sit inside your bra to catch this excess milk.

When you have a lot of milk building up, your breasts can feel full and sore – this is called engorgement. You may need to express a little milk if your breasts are feeling especially full and your baby doesn't need feeding at that moment to help you feel more comfortable.

If you're feeding a lot, your nipples can become quite sore, especially if your baby isn't latching as well as they could. There are lots of creams you can get to help, as well as nipple shields, but it's important to speak to your healthcare team, as cracked nipples can get infected. Another potential problem is blocked milk ducts, which can feel like a painful, hard lump and again should be checked out. If a blocked duct isn't dealt with, it can lead to inflammation and an infection called mastitis, which can make your breasts go hot and painful, and give you flu-like symptoms.

REBUILDING YOUR STRENGTH

It's usually advised to wait until after your postnatal check at six weeks before you start exercising again, but you shouldn't suddenly rush back into an intense programme. If you can, try to follow a plan designed for postpartum exercise. These tend to be tailored to build up slowly but steadily. If you feel any pain, you should stop and not try to push through. If you had a C-section, you will need to be even more careful so that you don't pull at the stitches. It may be several months before you can resume higher-impact activity.

It's best to start with gentle exercise, such as walking or swimming, which are low impact but will also start to build up your stamina and cardiovascular system. You may want to add in some yoga or Pilates – look for a class that is designed for postnatal women, as these will usually incorporate pelvic floor exercises as well as increasing strength. You can build muscle strength through weight training, but don't go back to lifting heavy weights too quickly as this can cause problems with your pelvic floor and core muscles. Start with very light weights, resistance bands or even bodyweight and increase from there.

Listen to your body and make sure that you're fuelling yourself with healthy and nutritious foods to give it the best chance of healing. ■

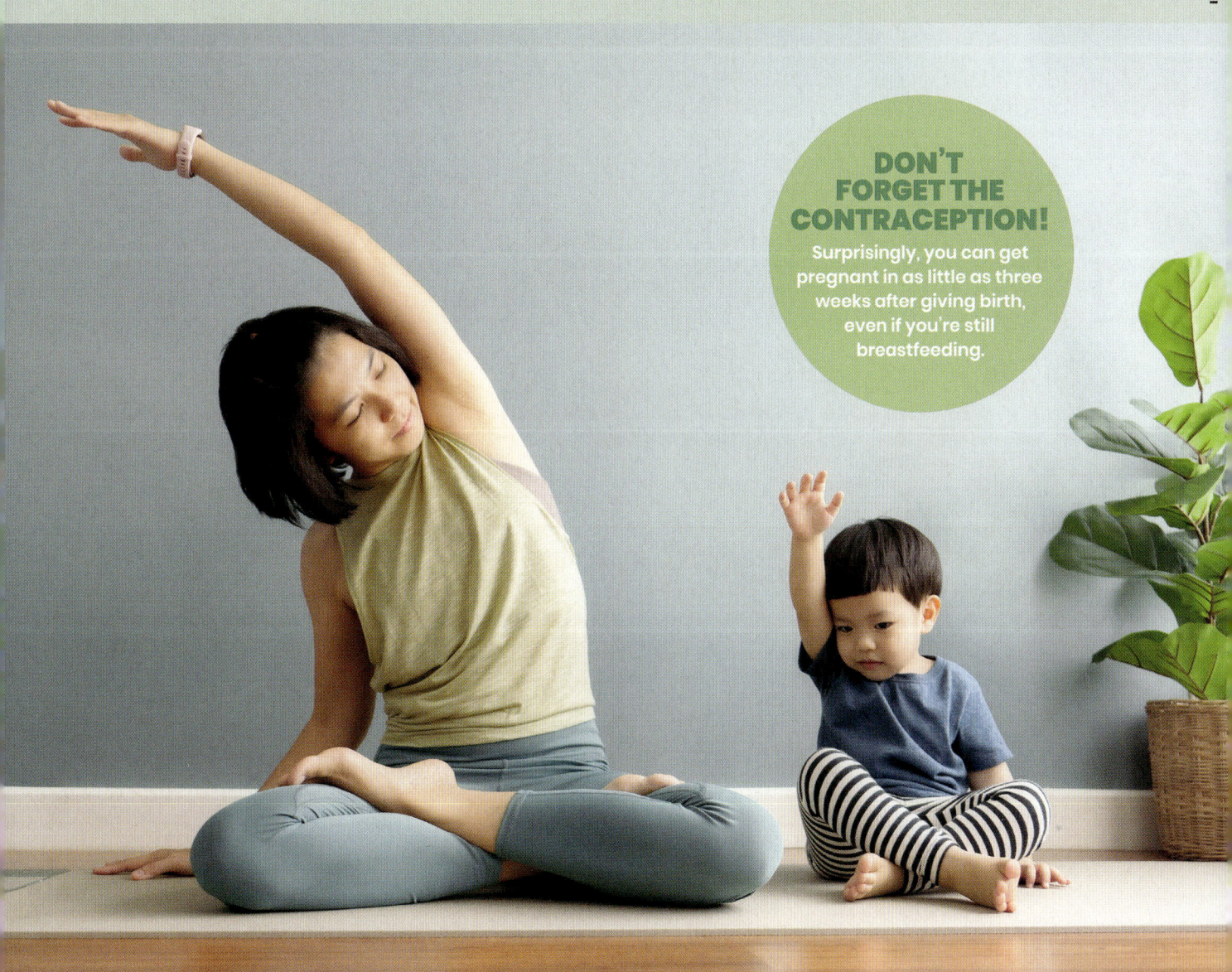

Postpartum Health

IMAGES Getty Images SOURCES NHS UK.

DON'T FORGET THE CONTRACEPTION!
Surprisingly, you can get pregnant in as little as three weeks after giving birth, even if you're still breastfeeding.

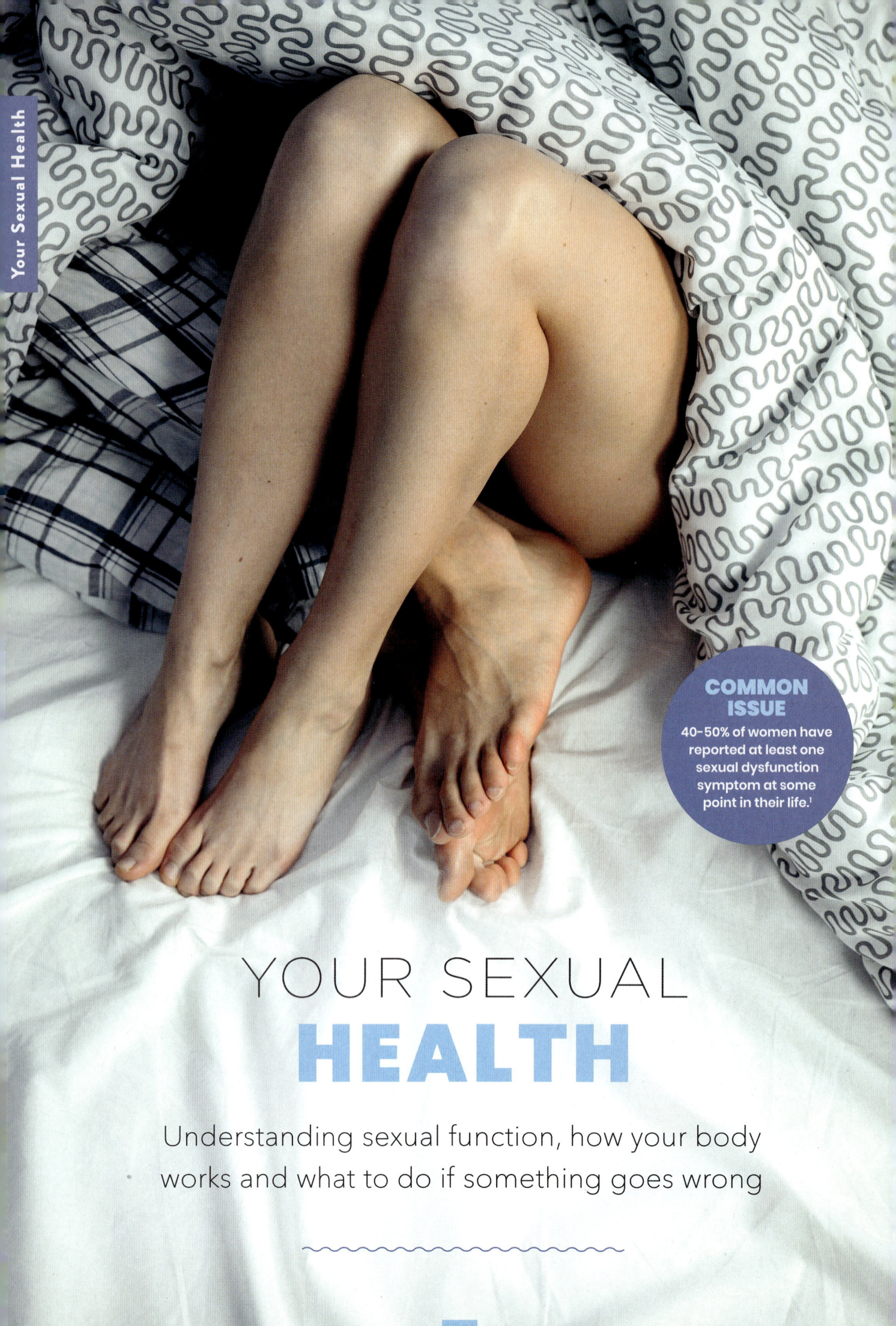

Your Sexual Health

COMMON ISSUE
40-50% of women have reported at least one sexual dysfunction symptom at some point in their life.[1]

YOUR SEXUAL
HEALTH

Understanding sexual function, how your body works and what to do if something goes wrong

Sexual function might not be a common topic of conversation among friends, but it's really important to understand your own sexual health, learn what's normal for you and know what to do when something isn't quite right. It shouldn't be embarrassing to talk about our body in this way, though stigma and societal norms can make the subject feel taboo. Knowledge is power, so learning about your sexual function can empower you to understand what's happening in your body, as well as help you to articulate any concerns you may have.

VAGINAL HEALTH

How much time do you spend thinking about your vaginal health? Probably not a lot, but being in good sexual health is an indication of good overall health. It means that you're able to have and enjoy pain-free sex with pleasure. It's also an important element in reproductive ability. Poor vaginal health can have an impact on your day-to-day life, your relationships and your self-esteem. Learning the symptoms and signs of problems with your vaginal health can mean that you catch and address any issues before they cause long-term concerns.

To clarify, the vagina is the muscular canal that leads from the vulva on the outside to the cervix at the neck of the womb. It is also known as the birth canal in the context of pregnancy and childbirth. The canal is quite stretchy and flexible. The wall lining has mucous membrane, which helps to lubricate and protect the canal. The lower third of the canal has a high concentration of nerve endings, which help with inducing pleasure during sex, as well as helping with the pain of childbirth. Surrounding the opening of the vagina are the labia majora (outer folds) and the labia minora (inner folds).

If your vagina is in good health, you shouldn't notice any pain or irritation. The canal should feel soft and flexible, rather than tight and strained (you can test this yourself by gently inserting a finger). The vagina produces a small amount of discharge to keep it healthy, which is normally clear or white. The consistency changes throughout your cycle, but it shouldn't have a strong or bad smell – if it does, this can be a sign of an infection.

> **"LEARNING ABOUT SEXUAL FUNCTION CAN EMPOWER YOU TO UNDERSTAND YOUR BODY"**

You don't need to do anything special to look after your vagina; it pretty much looks after itself. Your vagina has its own microbiome, made up of bacteria and other microorganisms, which work together in balance to keep your canal clean and healthy. Using any products can disrupt this delicate system, which can lead to infection, soreness, dryness and pain.

There are a lot of different conditions and health concerns that can impact your vaginal health. This includes inflammation, yeast infections, bacterial infections and sexually transmitted infections (STIs). It is possible for more serious problems to occur, such as vaginal cancer and vulvar cancer; both are very rare, but it's worth seeking medical advice if you have concerns, particularly around pain, itching, burning or unusual discharge.

STIs

Unprotected sex can put you at risk of a sexually transmitted infection

Nobody wants to have an STI – it's embarrassing to deal with, speak to partners about and seek medical assistance for. However, it's important that you do get infections treated as quickly as possible, so that they can't develop and cause more serious problems. It's something that is quite common – in the UK in 2023, there were more than 400,000 STIs diagnosed[2] – so any doctor or nurse you speak to is quite used to it and won't judge you in any way. Most infections are easily treatable and you can get advice from your usual doctor or a sexual health clinic. Symptoms to watch out for include unusual discharge, unusual bleeding, itching, inflammation, sores or warts, rashes, lumps or pain when urinating. Some STIs, like chlamydia, don't have any symptoms at all, but can cause serious health concerns if left untreated. For this reason, it's always best to have protected sex with a new partner, and consider a check-up at a sexual health clinic before choosing to have unprotected sex with a trusted partner.

▶ SEXUAL FUNCTION

One of the primary functions of the vagina is for sex. The process of sexual arousal prepares the vagina and vulva in a less obvious but equally significant way as it does for a man's penis. The nerve endings in the vagina are limited, but they do help with arousal when stimulated. However, it is the role of the clitoris that is most significant for arousal. When you first start getting excited, the vagina will produce more lubrication and extra blood will flow to the area. The labia will spread open to expose the external part of the clitoris, which in turn gets bigger in response to the increased blood flow. The internal part of the clitoris spans back into the body and is densely populated with nerve endings, which are what cause intense feelings of pleasure when stimulated. In response to stimulation, the clitoris swells in a similar way to the male erection. The vagina lengthens, while the opening contracts due to the increased blood flow. The labia also swell and can change colour to a deeper pink or red.

This process of arousal is what is achieved during foreplay, that is, manual stimulation of the vagina, vulva and clitoris before penetration. Many women also have other areas of the body that help with arousal, called erogenous zones. This can vary from person to person and can include the bottom, breasts, inner thighs or neck. There are more unusual areas that you might not have considered, such as the armpits, backs of the knees, feet, ears and stomach, so it's always worth experimenting to find out what you enjoy and what helps with arousal. Getting comfortable with your own body, through masturbation, can help you learn what feels good and what areas are particularly sensitive.

The peak of sexual arousal is orgasm. At this point, the clitoris is at its maximum size and sensitivity. An orgasm causes intense feelings of pleasure throughout the body, as well as muscle contractions through the vagina and pelvic region. Typically, one orgasm is made up of 15 or more contractions! Some women may have a female

TALKING TO A DOCTOR ABOUT SEX

It's not easy to address sexual health problems, so here are some tips

BE PREPARED
Write down your concerns, as this can make it easier for you to remember what you want to say in the moment, especially if you get distracted or embarrassed.

FIRST WORDS
The doctor won't know what's wrong, so you will have to broach the topic. You may wish to start off by saying something like, "I feel uncomfortable talking about this, but I'd like to discuss some sexual problems with you." This will open the conversation and the doctor can ask the right questions.

REQUEST A DOCTOR
You may prefer to speak to a female doctor, so if you do and it would make you more comfortable, make sure that you request this when making your appointment.

BE HONEST
Your doctor can't help if you're not honest with them. You need to be ready to answer questions that might be quite personal, but they are necessary for the doctor to get you the help you need.

ejaculation too, releasing clear liquid; it's perfectly normal and part of the experience. After orgasm, the vagina will naturally begin to relax, the blood flow will slow down and everything returns to its normal size and colour. It's not always easy to reach orgasm, as it relies on both mind and body being in the right state of arousal. Some women can only orgasm through clitoral stimulation, either on its own or combined with vaginal penetration. Again, it's about learning what you enjoy, on your own or with a partner, so that you have the best experience for yourself.

COMMON CAUSES OF SEXUAL DYSFUNCTION

There are many reasons and causes for physical sexual dysfunction. For example, hormone changes can have a big impact. In perimenopause and menopause, for example, it's not uncommon to experience vaginal dryness due to the dropping oestrogen levels, which can make penetrative sex more uncomfortable. Some medicines can impact on sexual function too, as can external influences like stress, mental-health concerns, illness and relationship problems.

Sometimes you can find it difficult to get physically aroused, mentally aroused or both. Things like drinking too much alcohol, recreational drugs, certain anti-depressants or not having enough sleep can make it physically difficult to feel aroused, even when stimulated. It can help to take the pressure off for a bit, giving you time to work on the underlying issues and have a bit of space before trying again (when you're ready). It might be that you need a little more time spent on foreplay, extra lubricant or a little experimentation to find a method that works for you.

> **"IT'S ABOUT LEARNING WHAT YOU ENJOY ON YOUR OWN OR WITH A PARTNER"**

Many women also have difficulty orgasming – it's more common than you might think! Issues might include not being able to orgasm at all, taking longer to orgasm or having fewer orgasms as you get older. Again, this can be linked to health conditions or medications, or, more rarely, if you've had surgical treatment in the pelvic area.

Another common reason for sexual dysfunction is pain, which can be just during sex or at all times. This means that it can be difficult or very uncomfortable to have penetrative sex. There are lots of different reasons for pain, from vaginal dryness to various infections and conditions. You can try using more lubrication, spending longer on foreplay to increase natural lubrication, or try a vaginal moisturiser.

However, if you are having any kind of new sexual dysfunction, especially without an obvious underlying cause, consider speaking to a doctor, who can give advice or run tests to find out more. ■

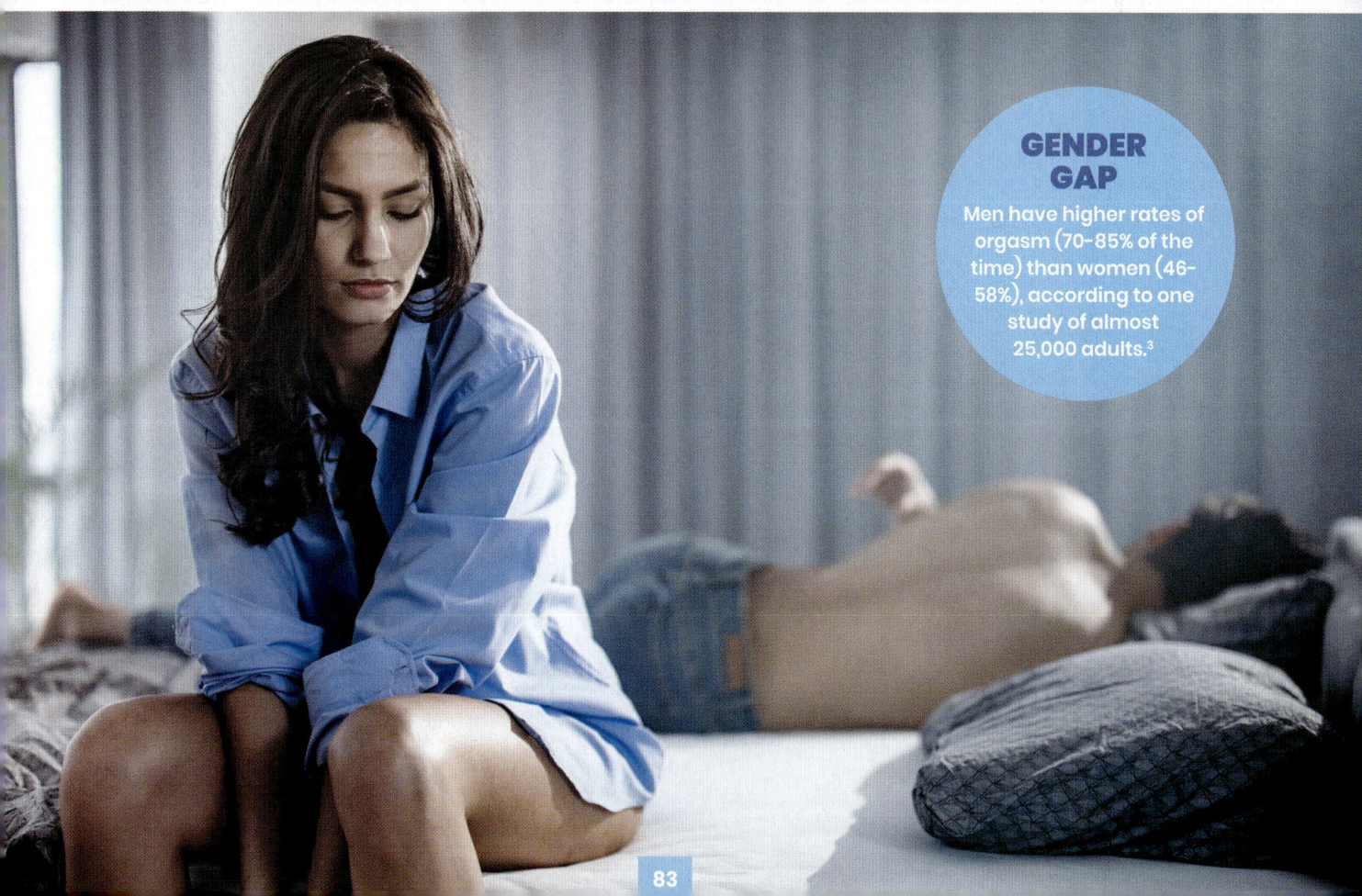

GENDER GAP
Men have higher rates of orgasm (70-85% of the time) than women (46-58%), according to one study of almost 25,000 adults.[3]

IMAGES Getty Images SOURCES [1] Prof. Rossella E Nappi et al. Female sexual dysfunction (FSD): Prevalence and impact on quality of life (QoL), 2016. [2] Gov.uk. [3] Amanda N Gesselman et al. The lifelong orgasm gap: exploring age's impact on orgasm rates. June 2024.

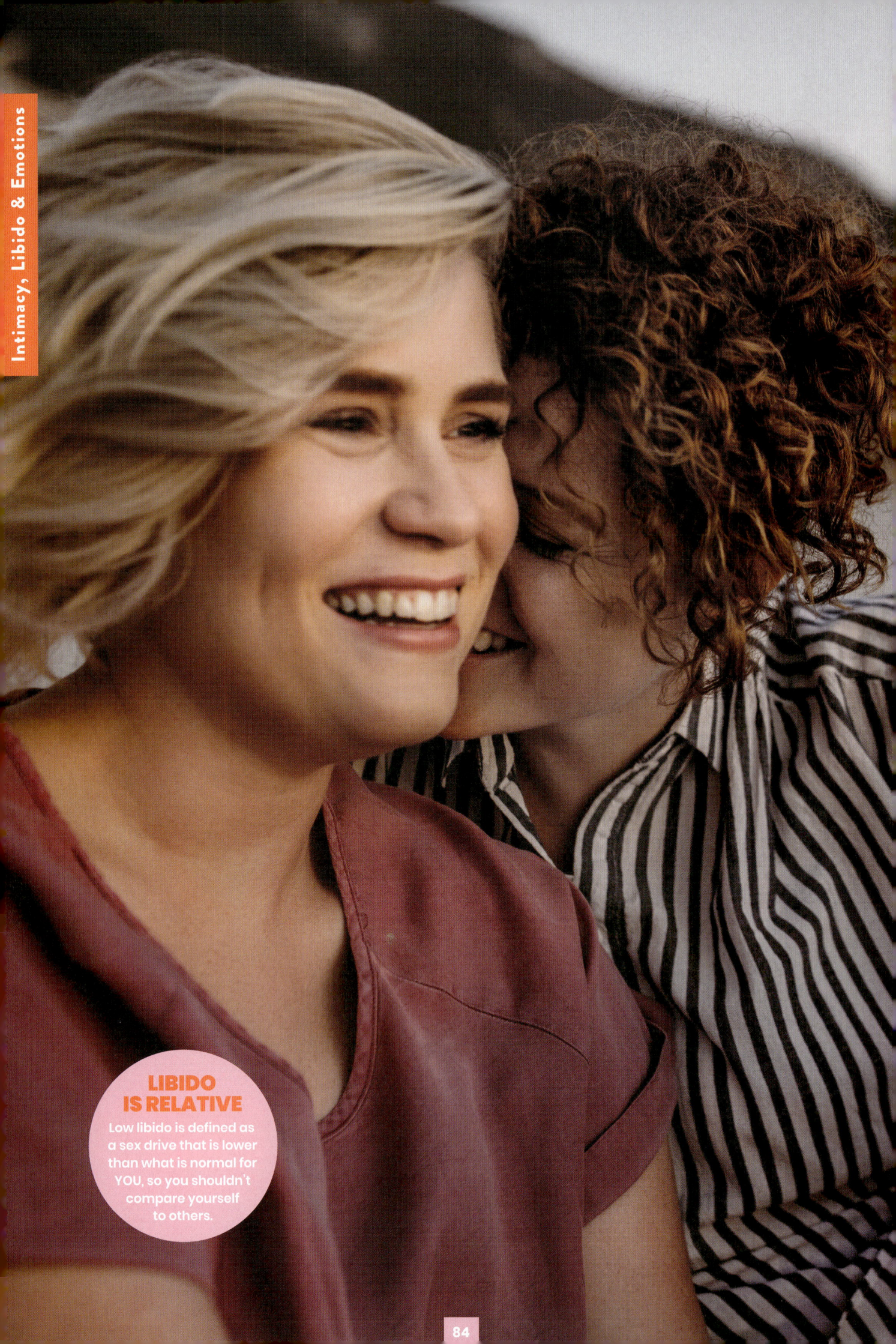

Intimacy, Libido & Emotions

LIBIDO IS RELATIVE
Low libido is defined as a sex drive that is lower than what is normal for YOU, so you shouldn't compare yourself to others.

INTIMACY, LIBIDO & EMOTIONS

Sex isn't just a physical act – your sexual health has a mental aspect too

Sex and intimacy mean different things to everyone. Things like desire, sex drive and emotions attached to sex are very personal. To understand your sexual health fully, it means learning more about the mental side of sex as well as the physical. Our desire and feelings towards sex will ebb and flow over our lifetime, and there are many reasons why we might feel less inclined at some points, but very enthusiastic at others.

EMOTIONS AND SEX

Attraction is a difficult concept to put into words. What is it that attracts us to another person? Sometimes it's a purely physical attraction, our body responding positively to the way someone looks, for example. It might be sexual attraction, where you're drawn to have sex with someone without needing a deeper connection. Or it could be an emotional attraction, where you're attracted to someone's personality and the way they connect with you.

Our body can pick up on lots of little cues, from speech to scent, from conversation to chemistry. Attraction can be instant or it can develop over time. As you build awareness of your own thoughts, feelings and physical reactions, you'll become more in tune with what you're attracted to and why. This innate sense of attraction is what draws us to sexual partners, helping to increase our desire for sex. One study suggests that there are intrinsic links between our desire for sex, our emotional pathways and our reproduction systems, fuelled by hormones.[1]

There is certainly an emotional element to having sex. After a positive sexual experience, you'll probably feel happy, relaxed, calm and satisfied, thanks to the release of certain hormones. And yet, despite the same physical response and the release of the same hormones, after a negative sexual experience you might have a different set of emotions, such as guilt, regret or embarrassment. For truly great sex, it takes our mental and physical sexual health to both be in the right place. That doesn't mean the same thing to everyone all the time. A casual sexual encounter can have just as much impact as regular sex within a long-term relationship, as long as you feel comfortable and have clear expectations.

Intimacy is more than just sex, so if you're looking to create a deeper connection with someone, then that goes far beyond the bedroom. It's about communication, affection, commitment and being present. That intimacy can carry through into sex too, deepening the experience and emotions you feel in a different way.

Ultimately, what you want from a sexual relationship and what you're comfortable with is what matters when it comes to your sexual health. If you're mentally in the mood and happy with the situation, then your physical responses will be heightened, leading to a better overall experience.

LIBIDO

Your libido is your desire for sex, otherwise called your sex drive. It's partly driven by ▶

hormones, mainly testosterone, which is produced in small amounts in the ovaries and the adrenal glands in the kidneys. It plays a part in arousal and your ability to orgasm, too, so it's an important hormone for overall sexual function. Testosterone levels in women will peak some time in your 20s, and then naturally decreases over time, in particular after menopause. Women who have a surgical or medical menopause will also see their testosterone levels drop rapidly.

Alongside testosterone, oestrogen and progesterone also play a role in sex drive. This can mean that your libido changes throughout the span of a menstrual cycle, as the levels of these fluctuate. For many women, it's something that you can track alongside your periods. There is often a peak near to ovulation, when oestrogen and testosterone levels are at their highest. This makes sense; at a base level, as humans, we want to reproduce, so our body increases desire to encourage procreation. You may also find that your sex drive naturally lessens after menopause, when you are no longer in your reproductive years, but that's not to say you can't boost it and continue to enjoy a healthy and fulfilling sex life.

However, libido isn't just a biological reaction. It is easily influenced by external factors. There are many lifestyle-related reasons why you might notice a drop in your libido. If you're not getting enough sleep, have a poor diet, drink too much alcohol, smoke or take drugs, then this can cause your sex drive to wane. Looking after your general health is important; when you're feeling well in yourself, you're more likely to have a desire for sex. And you may find that your sex drive takes a while to come back after pregnancy and childbirth. Long-term medical conditions can also impact your sex drive, such as obesity, diabetes and cardiovascular disease.

> **"THERE ARE MANY LIFESTYLE-RELATED REASONS FOR A DROP IN LIBIDO"**

Certain types of hormonal contraceptives may impact your sex drive, such as the contraceptive pill or implant. This can sometimes be a temporary side effect as you get used to the hormones, but if it continues and you're worried, you can always try a different form of contraception. Other medicines that can have an impact include those for hypertension or drugs that block the production of testosterone.

Your mental health can influence your libido, too. One of the symptoms of depression, for example, is a loss of sex drive due to feeling generally low, hopeless and unmotivated. Unfortunately, medicines that are commonly used to treat depression can also negatively affect your sex drive, so if this becomes a problem, you may be able to try a different type of antidepressant. Stress and anxiety are also big factors in your libido. When you're feeling overwhelmed, busy and run-down, you're in survival mode, which can prevent you from feeling desire for sex.

HOW TO BOOST LIBIDO

If you do notice a dip in your sex drive, there are methods you can try to give it a kickstart. First, it's

---

TALKING TO A PARTNER

It's important to be honest and share your feelings when it comes to sex

It can be hard to talk to a partner about sex, no matter how long you've been together. In a new relationship there may need to be discussions about likes and dislikes, honesty when something isn't working, and boundaries. In a long-term relationship, life changes can affect how you feel about sex – whether that's a lessening of libido, a loss of desire or side effects from other health conditions, for example. Even in the closest of relationships, bringing up the subject of sex can sometimes feel awkward, which could be due to worry that the other person won't understand what you're saying and take it as an attack on them personally. However, in any trusting relationship, open and honest communication is key – and it can lead to a better relationship and intimacy. It's best to have the chat in a neutral location and at a suitable time. It's a good idea to give them a heads up that you want to talk to them about sex, so they don't feel confronted. Be honest about your needs or the way you're feeling to start a gentle conversation. And remember, it's good to revisit your conversation, to check in on any changes as time goes by.

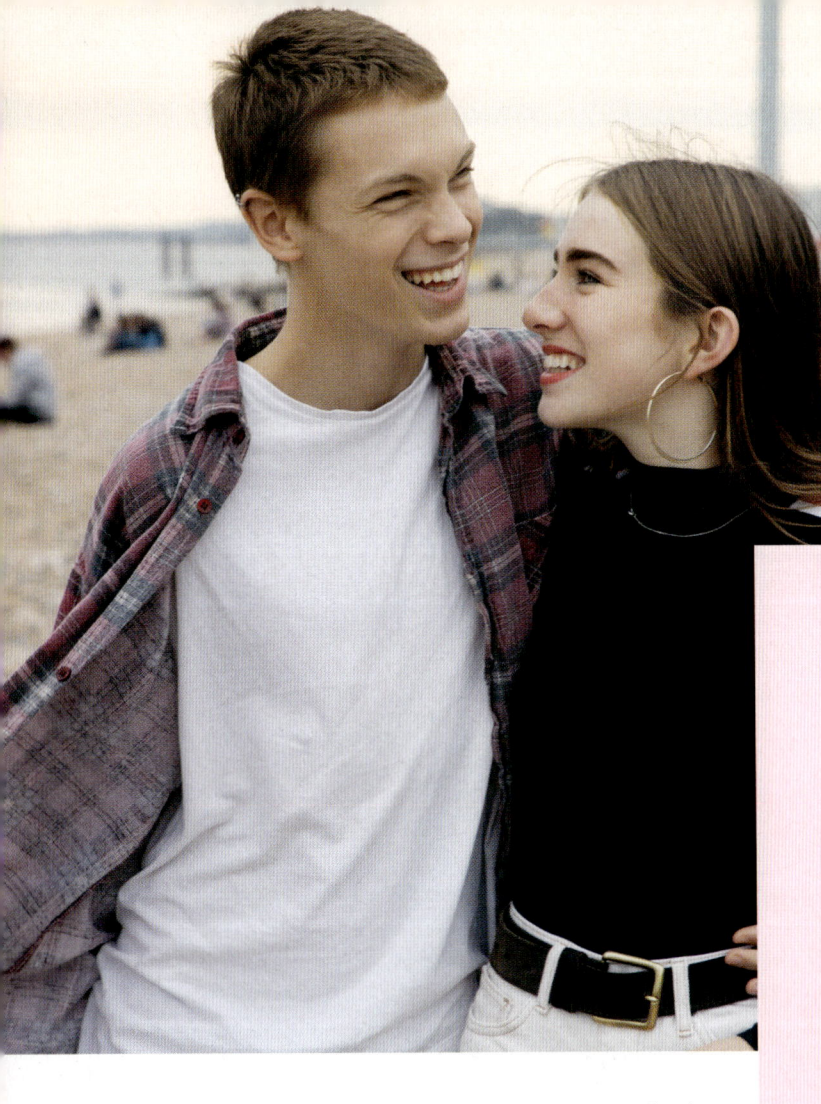

GOOD TO TALK
Chatting about sex with trusted friends can make you feel more comfortable and reassured with your own experiences.

worth eliminating any underlying health or medical reasons why this might be happening, such as the medicines you're taking or if you're suffering from another condition.

Otherwise, lifestyle interventions are the most effective way to boost your libido. This means making sure that you're getting enough high-quality sleep to boost your energy levels. Make sure that you're eating a well-balanced diet, with a particular focus on nutrient-dense fruits and vegetables. Exercise is important for encouraging blood flow and reducing stress, as well as helping you sleep, which can give your libido a surge. If you're under a lot of stress, you need to find ways to rest and relax, which could be things like stretching, yoga or meditation – although the best way to treat stress is to try to tackle the underlying cause and delegate where you can.

If your sex drive issues are linked to menopause, then HRT could be a solution, if you're able to take it. There are other medical treatments for low sex drive, such as bremelanotide (sold as Vyleesi™), which is touted as a female version of Viagra for use in pre-menopausal women. However, if your sex drive problems are rooted in a more emotional cause, then there are specific therapists who can help to unlock your thoughts, concerns and worries around sex, which can help to naturally boost your libido. These sessions can be attended alone or with a partner to try and get your sex life back on track to where you want it to be. ∎

MENTAL-HEALTH BENEFITS OF SEX

Having sex is good for your mental health! Here are some of the good bits

LOWERS STRESS LEVELS
Engaging in sexual activity can release endorphins, which can help to reduce stress and anxiety by making you feel calmer and more relaxed.

GOOD MOOD
Those same endorphins, as well as the production of dopamine, are responsible for giving you a mood boost and can help lift your spirits if you're feeling low.

DEEPER CONNECTIONS
Regular sex with a partner helps to build emotional connections and creates a more robust bond within a relationship.

BETTER SELF-ESTEEM
You might feel more confident in your own skin, which can help to boost your mental health.

SWEET DREAMS
Sex at night can help you both to drift off to sleep thanks to the release of oxytocin and prolactin, which are known to help you relax.

FEMALE HEALTH
CONCERNS

We look in more detail at some of the conditions that can impact women's health

ENDOMETRIOSIS

Endometriosis is a disease that impacts approximately 10% of women of reproductive age globally.[1] It's when tissue that is similar to the lining of the womb grows outside of the uterus in the pelvic area, causing inflammation and scar tissue to build up. This tissue can be found in the ovaries, the lining of the pelvis or the fallopian tubes, and occasionally around other pelvic organs, such as the bladder and bowel. These patches of tissue try to break down during your period like normal womb lining, but the bleed can't leave your body, which is what triggers symptoms. In very rare cases, endometriosis might be found outside the pelvic area, for example in the chest, which can cause pain in those areas.

Symptoms usually noticed around the time of a period include intense pain – far more so than normal period pain, and with a detrimental impact on your ability to do your normal daily activities. Periods may also be much heavier than is typical, soaking through a new pad or tampon in as little as an hour. There may also be pain when going to the toilet. It is often these menstrual cycle symptoms that lead to women seeking help and eventually a diagnosis, but there are symptoms and signs that can happen at other times before and after a period. This includes pain in the pelvic region, pain during or after sex, and fatigue.

Endometriosis can impact upon fertility too, making it harder to conceive, but it is usually possible to get pregnant. According to Endometriosis UK, it's estimated that 60-70% of those with endometriosis can get pregnant naturally.

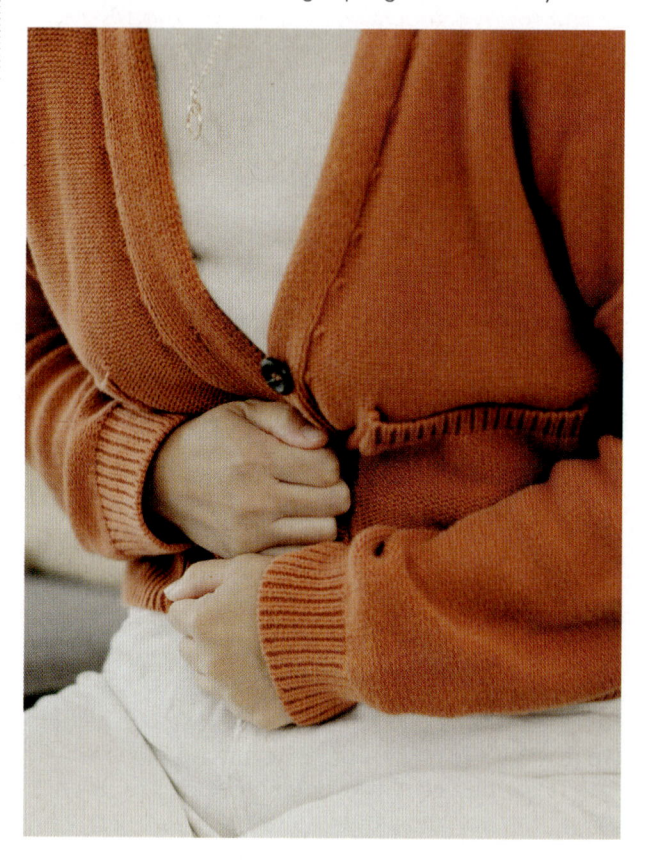

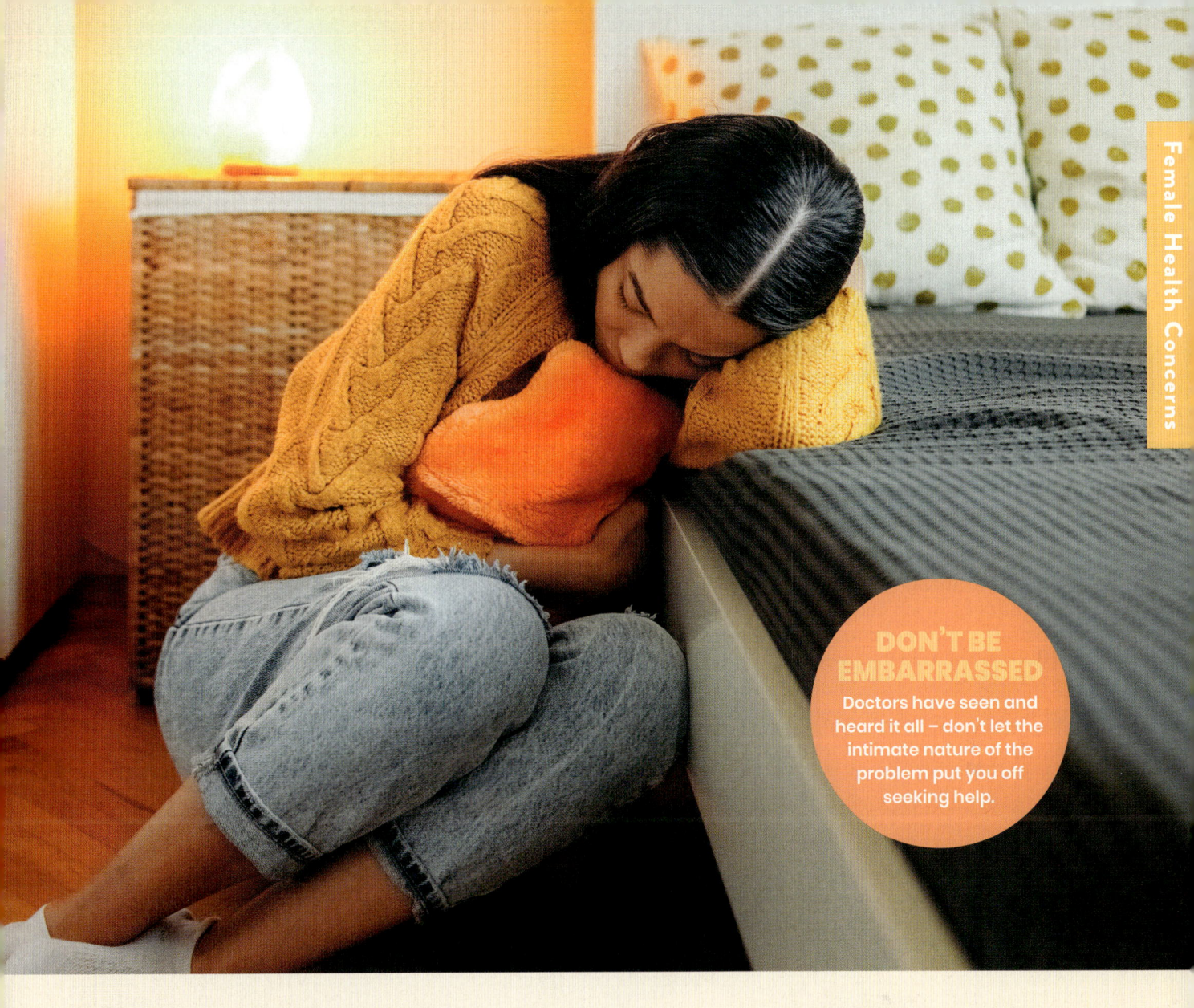

DON'T BE EMBARRASSED
Doctors have seen and heard it all – don't let the intimate nature of the problem put you off seeking help.

Having surgery to remove areas of endometriosis can help improve the chances of conceiving if the scar tissue is visible and superficial, though it may be less successful in improving fertility in cases of deeper endometriosis. Some women also find that their symptoms improve during pregnancy (although sadly they usually come back when periods do).

Symptoms can start from the first period in adolescence and last through until menopause. Anyone can develop endometriosis, and we don't yet know what causes it. Despite this, it can take a while to get diagnosed, as the symptoms can be similar to other conditions. Blood tests can help to confirm the presence or not of other conditions, and an internal ultrasound scan may be performed. Women with suspected endometriosis may also need a laparoscopy, which is when a camera is inserted through an incision near the belly button, to help gather more information for a diagnosis.

It is a chronic condition and there isn't a known cure, but there are ways to manage the symptoms. Some women find that using a hormonal contraceptive can help to manage pain and symptoms, and pain relief can also be used. However, if the areas of endometriosis are impacting significantly on day-to-day life, surgery may be needed to offer a longer-term solution. Areas of visible endometriosis can be removed, though more tissue can build up in the future. In more advanced cases, the womb, ovaries or affected parts of the bladder and bowel could be removed.

For many women, it's about learning to live with the symptoms and manage the long-term pain. There are various support groups that can help with this, including therapy sessions to help come to terms with the effects of the disease, as well as peer groups to talk to others with the same condition. In most cases, symptoms will taper off after menopause and often go away completely.

> **" ANYONE CAN GET ENDOMETRIOSIS. WE DON'T KNOW WHAT CAUSES IT AND IT CAN TAKE A WHILE TO GET DIAGNOSED "**

Female Health Concerns

PCOS

PCOS stands for polycystic ovary syndrome and is a hormonal condition that impacts how the ovaries work. It is the most common endocrine (hormonal system) condition in women. According to the World Health Organization, PCOS affects an estimated 6-13% of all reproductive-aged women globally. It usually begins in adolescence, but symptoms can vary over time and some women have no symptoms at all. Polycystic ovaries are often enlarged and form underdeveloped follicles that do not release an egg – they're not actually cysts, despite the name. Someone with PCOS might have irregular periods and excess levels of androgen (a male sex hormone, such as testosterone, though all women do produce small amounts of it), which can cause physical symptoms.

We don't know what causes PCOS specifically, but we do know that it is related to hormonal imbalances. It can run in families, so it may have a genetic element. It has been linked to insulin

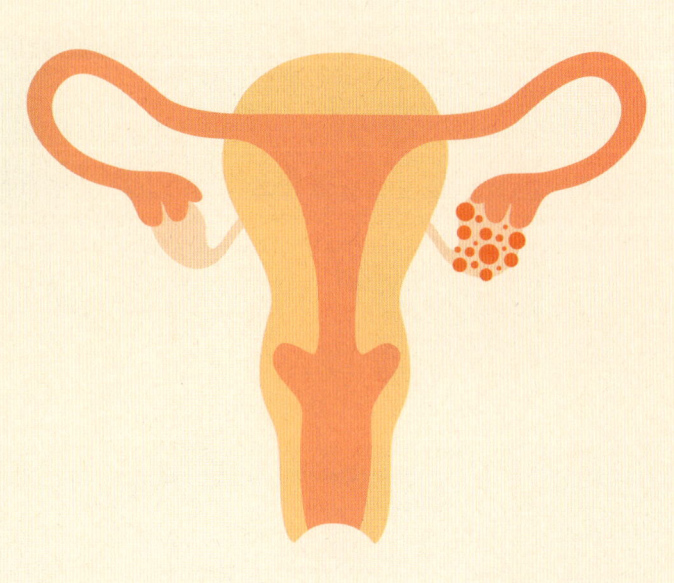

> **"SYMPTOMS VARY FROM PERSON TO PERSON"**

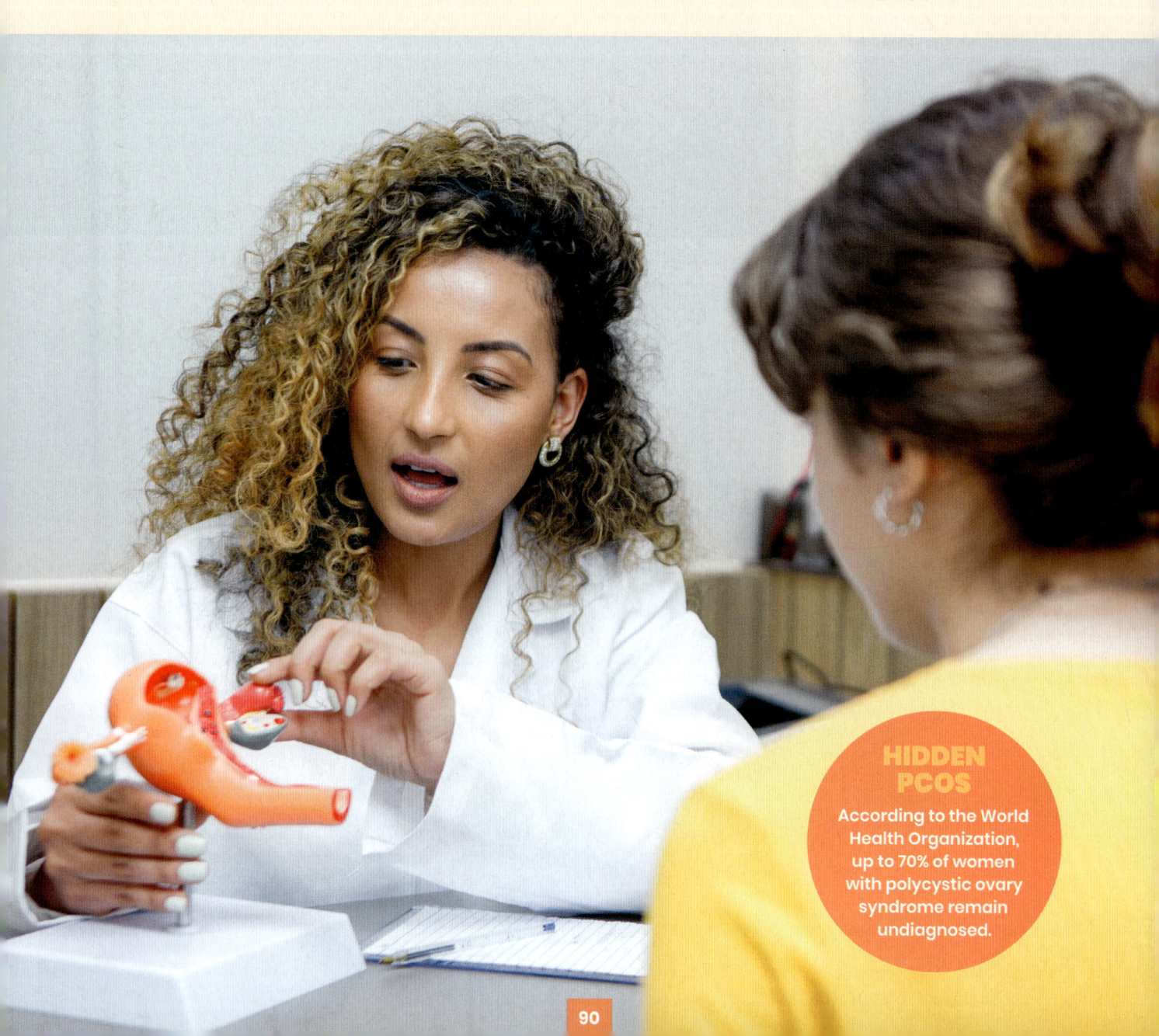

HIDDEN PCOS

According to the World Health Organization, up to 70% of women with polycystic ovary syndrome remain undiagnosed.

resistance, the hormone that controls blood sugar levels; when the body is resistant to insulin, it needs to produce more to try to bring blood sugar levels under control. High insulin levels can trigger the ovaries to produce too much testosterone and impact on the normal development of follicles during the menstrual cycle. Insulin resistance can also contribute to weight gain, which can worsen PCOS symptoms. Women with PCOS will often have high levels of testosterone, luteinising hormone and prolactin, but we don't yet fully understand why this happens.

Because of the link to insulin, PCOS increases the risk of developing type 2 diabetes. It can also impact on blood pressure and cholesterol, with high levels of these increasing the risk of heart disease and stroke. Weight gain due to PCOS can come with its own problems too, such as sleep apnoea. Women who have very irregular periods or don't have periods at all can have a higher, though still small, risk of developing endometrial cancer.

Symptoms vary from person to person, and they usually start from a woman's late teens to early 20s. One of the most obvious signs is that a woman has irregular periods or no periods at all. This leads to fertility problems – PCOS is one of the most common reasons for female infertility. Other symptoms are triggered by the hormonal imbalances including excessive hair on the face, chest or back, weight gain, hair loss or thinning, and oily skin problems, such as acne. These physical symptoms can be hard to cope with, and some women with PCOS struggle with their self-esteem and confidence as a result.

PCOS is a chronic condition with no cure, so treatment aims to manage the symptoms. Lifestyle changes to encourage a healthy weight are usually advised, as this can lessen symptoms. Sometimes the contraceptive pill is used to help create a regular cycle of periods, which means that the womb lining doesn't build up too much, lowering the risk of endometrial cancer. There are also treatment options for those struggling with fertility to encourage ovulation to take place; treatments for hair growth and hair loss; as well as medication for any side effects like hypertension or high cholesterol levels. Some women will opt for IVF treatment to help with fertility if medication doesn't help to regulate ovulation. There is also a surgical procedure called laparoscopic ovarian drilling (LOD), which can help with fertility problems by destroying the tissue that is producing androgens, restoring normal hormonal balance.

VULVOVAGINAL HEALTH

There are some health conditions that can impact your vagina and vulva

THRUSH
Thrush is a very common yeast infection that causes a white vaginal discharge, itching around the vulva and vagina, and soreness when having sex or going to the toilet. It's easy to treat with antifungal medication, which is usually an oral tablet or a vaginal pessary, and creams to reduce the itching.

BARTHOLIN'S CYST
These cysts are small fluid-filled sacs just inside the opening of the vagina. They don't normally cause problems unless they grow large, which can cause pain and swelling. If the cyst gets infected, it can become red and hot, and you may get a temperature. They don't usually need treatment, but if they are painful you can soak in warm water to relieve the pain and use painkillers.

VAGINITIS
This is soreness and swelling around the vaginal opening. You may have itching, soreness, unusual vaginal discharge, dryness, light bleeding and sore skin. It can occur as the result of another condition, such as thrush, a sexually transmitted infection like chlamydia, or a skin condition like eczema. It can also occur around menopause due to the hormonal changes.

VULVAL PAIN
This is non-specific pain that occurs in the vulva. Sometimes the pain is constant, but it can also come and go, and it may worsen during sex or when using the toilet. You may be referred to a specialist to help find appropriate treatment depending on the triggers. ▸

FIBROIDS

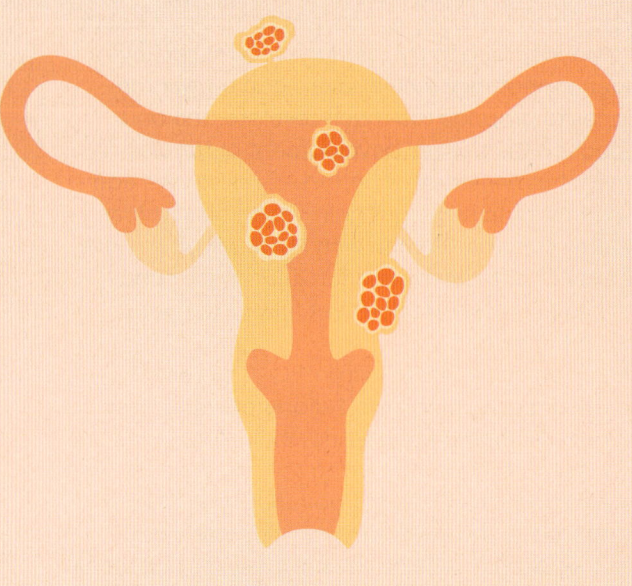

Fibroids are a type of growth within the womb; women can have more than one fibroid, and they can be different sizes. These growths are non-cancerous, made up of muscle and tissue. They are very common – it's thought that about eight in ten women get them,[2] but as they don't cause symptoms in around two-thirds of cases, most of us wouldn't even know that we have them. They grow slowly during our reproductive years, but after menopause they usually stop growing and begin to shrink again.

There are different types of fibroids, depending on where they grow and how large they have the potential to become. The most common type is an intramural fibroid, which develops in the muscular wall of the womb. A subserosal fibroid develops outside the wall of the womb and into the pelvis – these can grow very large. Finally, a submucosal fibroid can develop within the muscle layer under the womb lining, growing into the cavity of the womb. Sometimes fibroids are attached to the womb via a narrow section of tissue; these are called pedunculated fibroids.

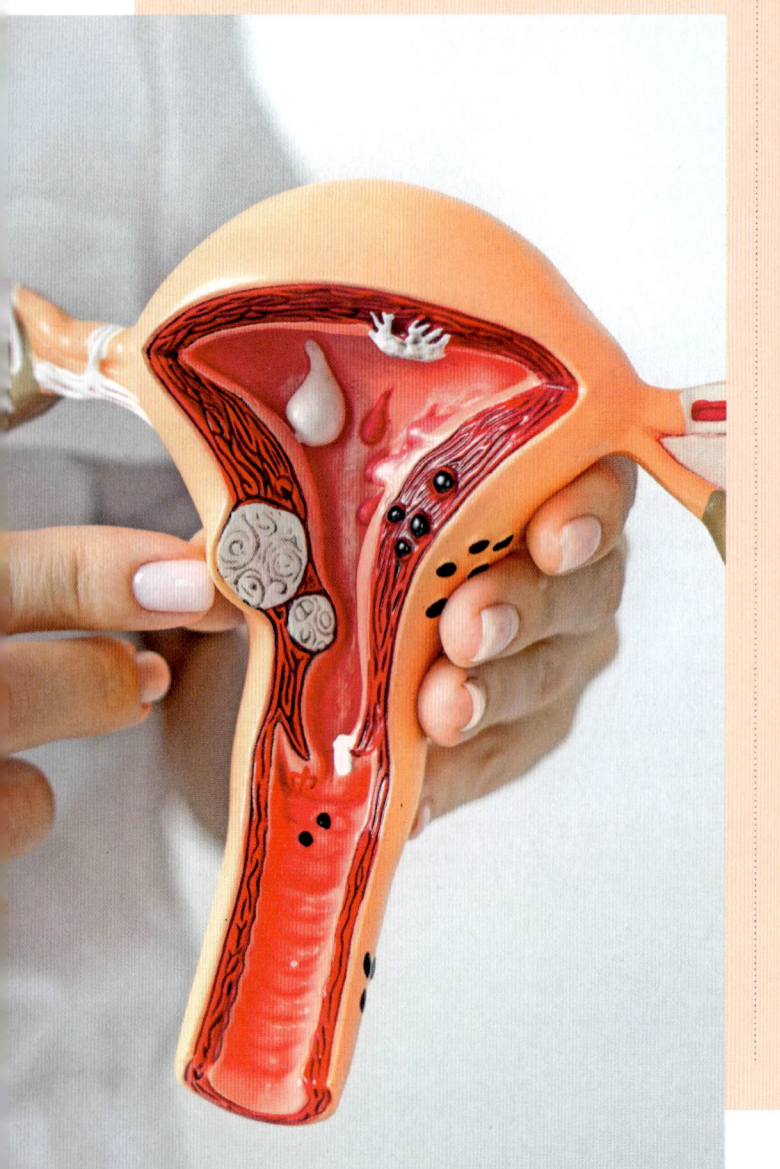

Anyone can develop a fibroid, though there is a slightly higher risk in women of African-Caribbean origin and in women who are overweight. Having children can lower the risk of developing fibroids. It's thought that they are caused by oestrogen, due to the fact that they grow during the reproductive years and shrink after menopause, but the exact cause is unknown.

For the one in three women[3] who do have symptoms, these can include heavy and/or painful periods, abdomen pain, lower back pain, constipation, a frequent need to urinate and pain during sex. These symptoms can be linked to a number of female health conditions, so they don't always mean fibroids. The presence of fibroids can be confirmed with an ultrasound scan.

As most fibroids don't cause symptoms, they don't necessarily need treatment. However, if they are having an impact on daily life, there are options. There are medicines that can help reduce heavy periods, including an LNG-IUS, which is a plastic T-shaped device that is inserted into the womb to release a hormone that can help control the growth of the womb lining, leading to lighter periods. Some contraceptive pills can also help to reduce heavy and painful periods, as can progestogen (either orally or via injection). There are medicines that can actively reduce the size of the fibroids, which may lessen the symptoms. In more extreme cases, it might be necessary to perform surgery to remove the fibroids or the womb.

TRACK SYMPTOMS

When it comes to diagnosis, it can be helpful if you keep a diary of your symptoms alongside your cycle.

ADENOMYOSIS

Adenomyosis is a condition that can impact any woman in their reproductive years – however, it is more common over the age of 30 and in women who have given birth. The lining of the womb starts to grow into the womb's walls, causing symptoms. It's estimated to affect around one in ten women in the UK and up to one in five women globally, but not everyone with adenomyosis has symptoms. There is no known cause.

> **"IT CAN IMPACT ON FERTILITY, THOUGH MANY WOMEN STILL GET PREGNANT NATURALLY"**

Those who do have symptoms will likely have painful and heavy periods during menstruation. Symptoms that can happen at any time include pain during sex, bloating or fullness in the stomach, and pelvic pain. These symptoms mirror those of many other female health conditions, so it's not always obvious that it's adenomyosis causing the problem. It is similar to endometriosis, where tissue similar to the womb lining grows in other places. Some women have both endometriosis and adenomyosis at the same time, but they are two different diseases.

It can be difficult to diagnose, as the excess growth is within the muscular walls of the womb. A doctor might first want to rule out other conditions. Initial tests may include a physical examination of your pelvis, as well as an internal check-up of the vagina and cervix. You may also get a pelvic ultrasound scan or MRI to look at the area in some more detail.

Treatment is designed to relieve the symptoms, which can include using hormonal contraception or an IUS (hormonal coil) to help manage pain and heavy periods. There are other medicines too, such as tranexamic acid, which helps to control bleeding, and anti-inflammatory drugs. If these options don't work, then it may need a surgical intervention, which can remove the lining of the womb (endometrial ablation) or the womb itself (hysterectomy). Otherwise, if symptoms are not too severe, you may be able to use a heat pad or painkillers to help with pelvic pain.

Adenomyosis can impact on fertility and pregnancy, though many women can get pregnant naturally with the condition. There have been recent studies that have shown a slight reduction of success of IVF in women with adenomyosis if they have been unable to conceive naturally.[4]

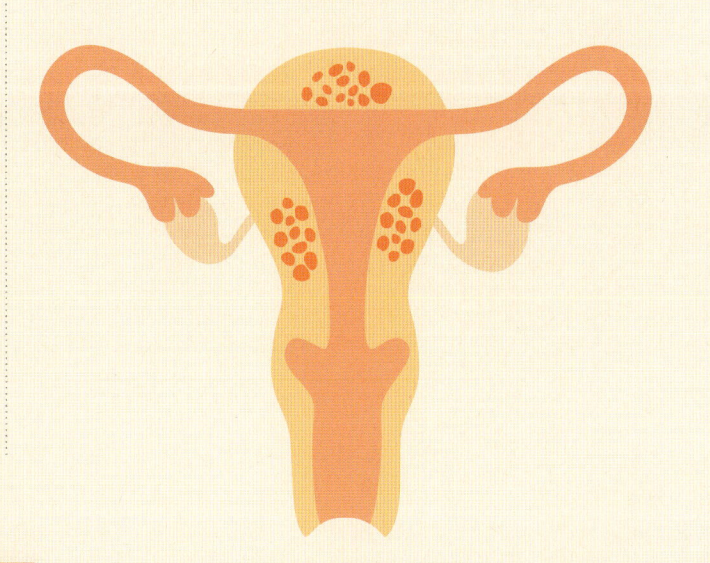

GYNAECOLOGICAL CANCERS

We look at the five main cancers of the reproductive system that can impact women, and their early warning signs

WOMB CANCER

Womb cancer (or uterine cancer) is a cancer that develops in the cells of the womb. Most cases of womb cancer are in the endometrium, the lining of the womb, so sometimes it will be called endometrial cancer. The cancerous cells are usually found in the glandular tissue, which means they are adenocarcinoma – this is the most common type of womb cancer. This is usually a 'type 1' endometrial cancer, which is linked to having excess oestrogen in the body. They are usually quite slow-growing and less likely to spread, meaning that if it's caught early, treatment is considered curative.

There are other types of womb cancer that are far less common, such as serous carcinoma and clear cell carcinoma. These also develop in the lining of the womb, but are classified as 'type 2' endometrial cancers, which means that they are not linked to excess oestrogen, making them faster-growing and more likely to spread. Another rare type of womb cancer is uterine sarcoma, also a type 2 cancer, which develops in the muscle layer of the womb rather than the lining and requires different treatment.

Symptoms of womb cancer include heavy or persistent bleeding between periods, unusual pink discharge, or bleeding after menopause. Some women may also have pain in their stomach, bloating or swelling, a change in bowel or bladder habits, and a newly developed cough. All these symptoms can be a sign of other, less serious conditions, like endometriosis and fibroids. So, while it is incredibly important to get checked out and find the underlying cause so it can be treated, try not to worry too much if you notice these symptoms, as womb cancer is the worst-case scenario. Early detection is key, as this can make it quicker and easier to treat, with a greater chance of success. In England, 90% of women with stage 1 womb cancer will survive for five years or more after diagnosis.[1]

Your first step is to speak to a doctor and be clear about your symptoms. It's useful if you can make a note of any bleeds, how heavy they were, and when they happened, as well as any other symptoms. This can help you to stay on track and make sure you cover everything. You'll usually be referred to a gynaecologist for a further check-up, which might include blood tests, an ultrasound scan or a biopsy of the affected area. You may also need more detailed scans such as a CT or MRI.

If you are diagnosed with womb cancer, you'll usually be given a stage, which means how advanced it is and whether it has spread beyond the womb lining. The main treatments are surgery to remove your womb and cervix, ovaries and fallopian tubes (a hysterectomy). For some women with low-risk womb cancer, this might be all the treatment that is needed. In premenopausal women, there may be an option to keep your ovaries. Higher-risk or more advanced womb cancers may need chemotherapy or radiotherapy, as well as potentially hormone treatments. ▶

> "IN ENGLAND, 90% OF WOMEN WITH STAGE 1 WOMB CANCER WILL SURVIVE FOR FIVE YEARS OR MORE"

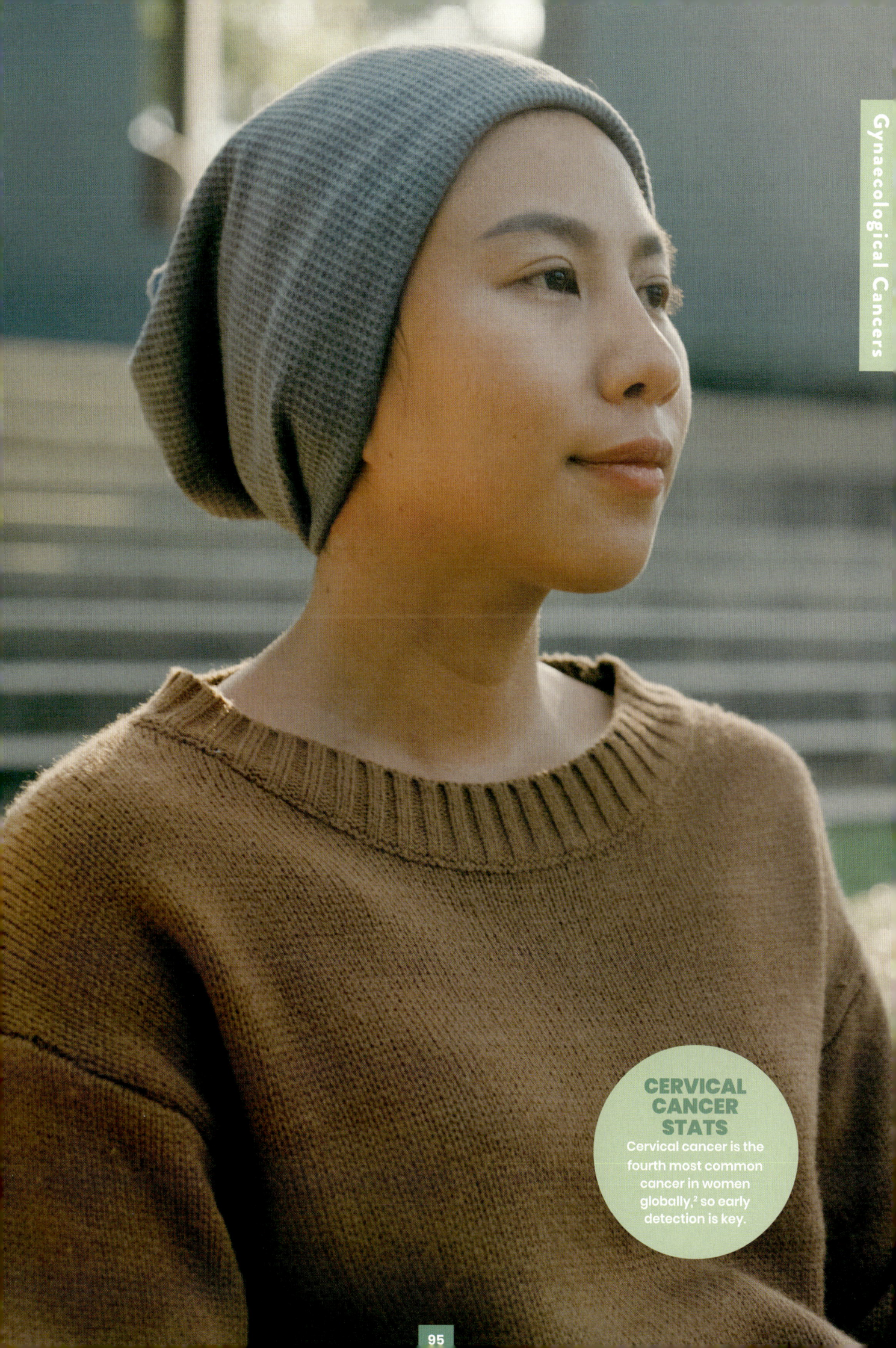

Gynaecological Cancers

CERVICAL CANCER STATS
Cervical cancer is the fourth most common cancer in women globally,[2] so early detection is key.

OVARIAN CANCER

Ovarian cancer is when abnormal cells develop in your ovary, which can then spread into the surrounding tissue and organs. There are different types of ovarian cancer. The most common is called epithelial ovarian cancer – it accounts for about 90% of all ovarian cancer cases. The cancer is found in the layer around the ovary. Even within epithelial ovarian cancer there are different sub types, the most common of which is called high-grade serous, which usually starts in the fallopian tube (called fallopian tube cancer) and spreads to the ovary where it grows. There is also primary peritoneal cancer (PPC), which starts in the lining on the inside of the stomach, called the peritoneum, and it is rare. The cells are the same as the most common type of ovarian cells, so it is treated in the same way as ovarian cancer. It mostly impacts people over the age of 60, and it's thought that the cancer starts in the cells at the end of the fallopian tube, before spreading to the peritoneum where it grows. Other types of epithelial ovarian cancer include endometroid and clear cell, which can both be linked to having endometriosis; low-grade serous, which is rare, slow-growing and more often diagnosed in younger people; and mucinous, which is also rare and difficult to diagnose.

Symptoms of ovarian cancer include pain in your abdomen, swelling and bloating, loss of appetite, changes in bowel and bladder habits, fatigue, weight loss, nausea and vaginal bleeding. These symptoms can indicate many other health conditions, so it's important to go to a doctor to rule out possible causes. These symptoms can also be linked to having ovarian cysts, which are not usually cancerous, and may go away without treatment.

In order to test for ovarian cancer, your doctor may examine your abdomen, do a pelvic exam (including an internal vaginal check) or do blood tests. If you are referred to a specialist, then you may have an ultrasound scan, a CT scan or a biopsy. When your blood is tested, you may be checked for CA125, which is a protein that is found in the blood, usually in low levels. Raised levels can indicate ovarian cancer in some cases, but it's not completely reliable on its own. Caught early, ovarian cancer can be treated, and at stage 1, 95% of women survive for five years or more.[1]

The main treatment plans for ovarian cancer are surgery and chemotherapy. Surgery removes the ovaries, fallopian tubes, the womb and the cervix to try to remove as much cancer as possible. For women who might want to have a baby in the future, it may be possible, if the cancer is low grade and low stage, to only remove the affected ovary and fallopian tube, leaving the rest intact. Radiotherapy or hormone treatment might also be used as part of your treatment plan.

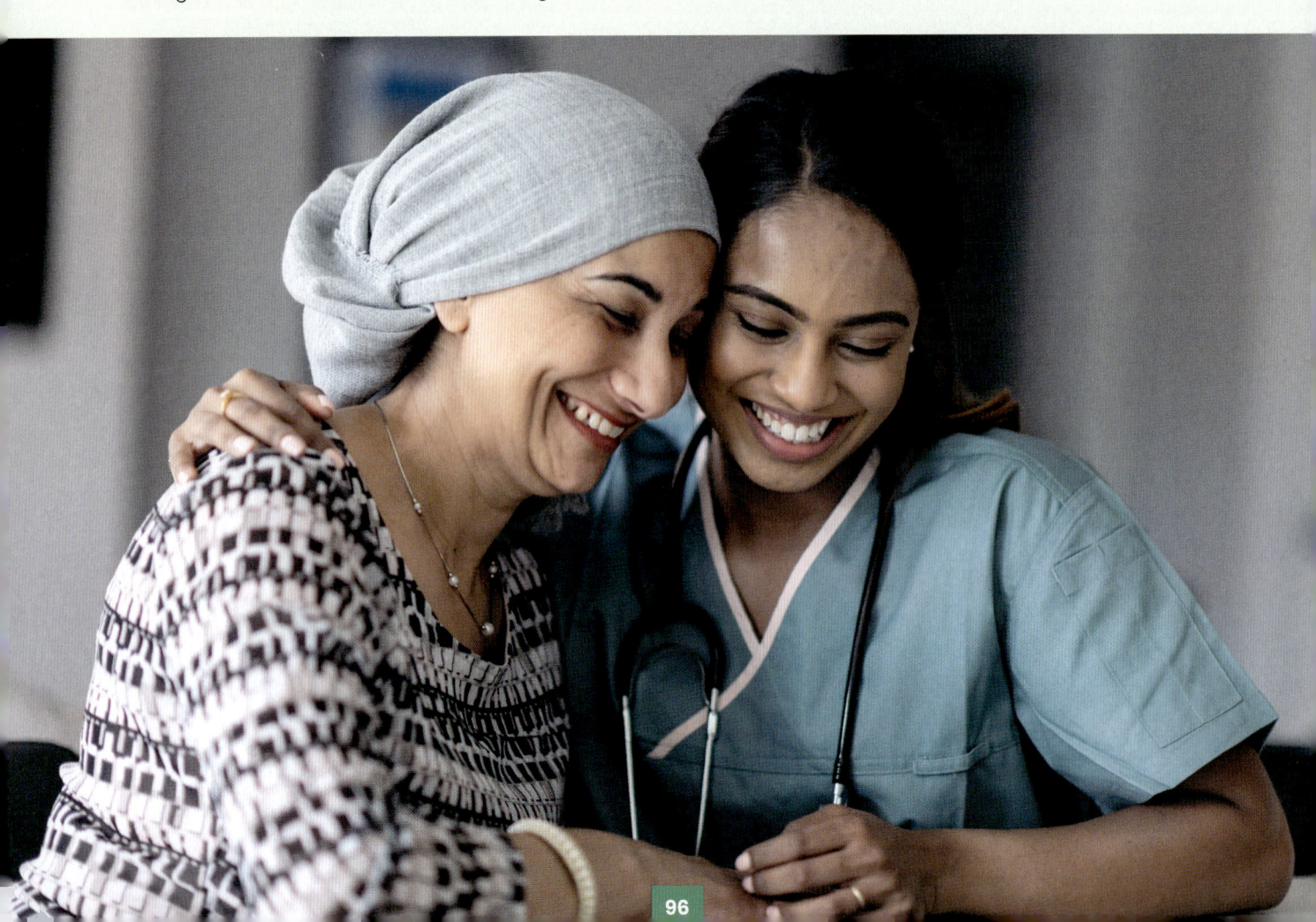

CERVICAL CANCER

Cervical cancer starts in the lining of the cervix, which is where a tumour develops. It can spread into the surrounding tissue and to other areas of the body. It is the most prevalent of all the gynaecological cancers and more common in women in their early 30s. The main cause of cervical cancer is a long-lasting infection of a certain type of HPV. HPV infection is very common, but most people's immune systems clear the infection.

Caught early, cervical cancer can be treated and there is a higher level of success. However, early cervical cancer doesn't have any symptoms, and by the time symptoms are detected, it may be at a more advanced stage. Symptoms include unusual bleeding, pain during sex, unusual discharge and pain in the pelvis. Because of the fact that early cervical cancer doesn't have symptoms, it's very important to be up-to-date with your cervical screening checks (sometimes also called a smear test or PAP smear). These screenings can detect the presence of high-risk HPV. If your sample shows that HPV is present, then further tests are done on the sample to see if there any cell changes. Not all cell changes will develop into cancer, but by detecting them at a very early pre-cancerous stage it means that they can be removed. There is now an HPV vaccine that can be given to young girls, which can protect against high-risk HPV, but it does not replace the need to also have regular cervical screenings.

> **"CAUGHT EARLY, CERVICAL CANCER CAN BE TREATED WITH A HIGHER LEVEL OF SUCCESS"**

HPV VACCINE
The HPV vaccine, when offered to girls aged 12-13 years old, may prevent up to 90% of cervical cancers.[1]

Tests for cervical cancer include internal and external examinations, blood tests or other scans. You may also need to have a colposcopy, which looks at the cervix in more detail, and biopsies may be taken. Caught early, cervical cancer can be treated and at stage 1, 95% of women survive for five years or more[1] – which is why cervical screening can be lifesaving.

In early-stage cervical cancer, which means that it is isolated to the neck of the womb or just into the top of the vagina, it can be treated with surgery to remove the womb and cervix. Those who might still want to have children and have stage 1 cancer may be able to have a radical trachelectomy, which aims to remove most of the cervix but leave enough to be able to be able to carry a baby, though there are no guarantees. You may also need chemoradiotherapy, which is a combination of chemotherapy and radiotherapy at the same time. The radiotherapy will be both external and internal (the latter is called brachytherapy). More advanced cases of cervical cancer may need different types of surgery (depending on where it has spread), chemoradiotherapy, or chemotherapy and radiotherapy separately, and immunotherapy. ▶

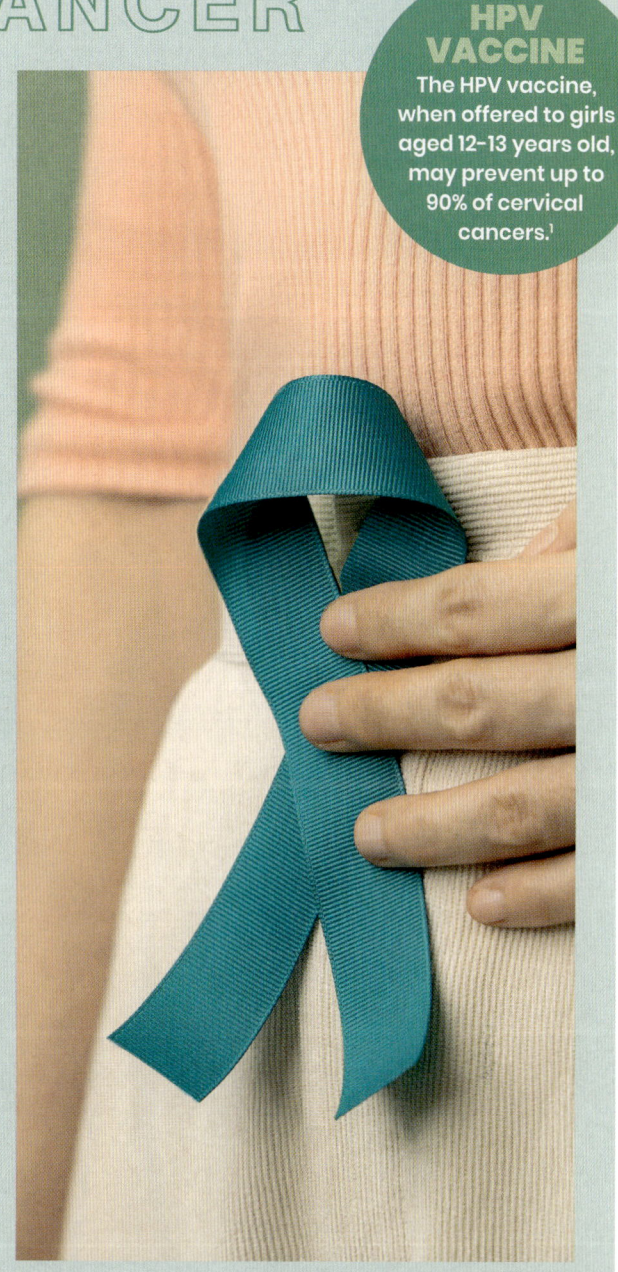

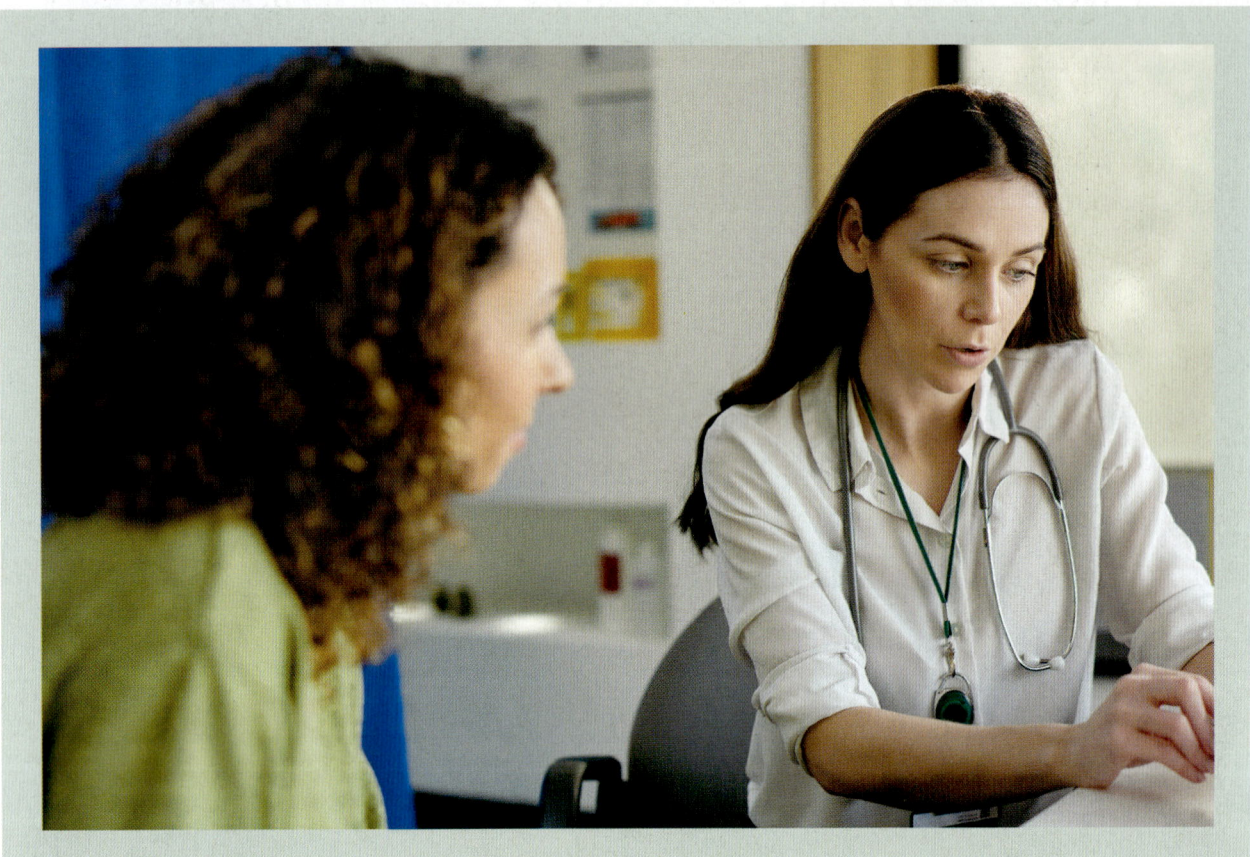

VULVAL CANCER

Vulval cancer is a female cancer that starts in any part of the vulva, most often in the inner or outer labia. Cancers in this area normally develop gradually. Some people have abnormal cells in the vulva that can be detected. These abnormal cells – called vulval intraepithelial neoplasia (VIN) – have the potential to develop into cancer, so they are sometimes called pre-cancerous, but they do sometimes go away on their own. If VIN is found early enough, then the abnormal cells can be treated before they have the chance to develop into anything more severe. Not all vulval cancers start in this way, so it's important to be aware of the symptoms.

Vulval cancer is rare, though the risk does increase slightly as you get older. The majority of cases are found in older women over the age of 75. In the UK, there are around 1,400 cases per year. The main symptoms include an open sore or growth on the skin of the vulva, persistent itching, bleeding, pain, a mole that changes shape or colour, a lump or swelling, or burning when you pee. These symptoms are also relevant for VIN, so if you notice any of these, you should speak to your doctor to be checked. Some of these symptoms also overlap with the symptoms for thrush, which is very common, and will clear up with treatment. Many of us don't check our vulva for changes regularly, but it is worth doing a self-examination each month between your periods. It can be embarrassing to discuss symptoms that impact your vulva with a doctor, which can be why some cases go undetected in the early stages, but it is very important to be checked as soon as possible.

Tests for vulval cancer start with a vulval examination. There may also be an internal vaginal examination to check your pelvis and abdomen. If you are referred to a specialist, then you may have a vulvoscopy and colposcopy to have a better look at the area, blood tests and scans. You will likely have a biopsy taken if anything is found that needs checking.

If you are found to have VIN, the first treatment may be a cream called imiquimod, which activates the immune system to attack and destroy abnormal cells. If you have a large area of VIN, you may need surgery to remove the affected skin and some of the surrounding area.

When it comes to vulval cancer, you will almost certainly need this surgery to remove part of the vulva. In very rare cases, the whole vulva may need to be removed. It may also be possible to have reconstructive surgery to rebuild the vulva. During surgery, lymph nodes from the groin will be taken and tested to see if the cancer has spread, in which case, radiotherapy and/or chemotherapy might also be needed.

VAGINAL CANCER

Vaginal cancer is very rare – globally, it accounts for fewer than 20,000 cases annually. In the UK, only about 250 women a year are diagnosed, mostly older women aged over 75 years old.[1] It is a cancer that starts in the vagina. Usually, the cancer starts in one of the tissue layers inside the vagina. There are different types of tissue, including the epithelial tissue, which is made up of squamous cells, and connective tissue, which is made up of muscle, lymph vessels and nerves. Most vaginal cancers will start in the squamous cells, called squamous cell carcinomas. Very rarely, the cancer will start in the gland cells, which is called adenocarcinoma. Even more rarely, cancer can develop in the connective tissue layer, called sarcomas. There are also lymph nodes in the groin, which is usually the first place that any cancer cells that break off from a tumour will go to, and from there may spread to other parts of the body. If cancer is found in the vagina, it could be because it has spread there from other areas as a secondary location. The primary cancer might be the cervix, vulva, bowel or womb, and this is not the same as having vaginal cancer.

Symptoms including bleeding between your periods or after menopause, bleeding after sex, unusual or pink discharge, pain during sex and a palpable lump or growth. In the early stages there may be no symptoms at all. It may be picked up during a routine cervical screening if the doctor notices any unusual lumps. These symptoms are also indicative of many other health conditions, so these need to be ruled out first. Given that vaginal cancer is so rare, a different underlying cause is far more likely. Women who have had a hysterectomy previously can still get vaginal cancer.

Testing for vaginal cancer can include a physical external and internal examination, blood tests, a colposcopy, a vaginal biopsy and other detailed scans. Some women may have vaginal intraepithelial neoplasia (VAIN), which means that abnormal cells are found in the lining of the vagina. This is not cancer, but sometimes these changes can develop into cancer; most of the time, VAIN won't develop into cancer. Women with high-grade or high-risk VAIN may be offered treatment to remove the abnormal cells.

Treatment for vaginal cancer includes surgery and radiotherapy. Surgery can include removal of the cancer area and a margin around it, the complete removal of the vagina (vaginectomy), or a radical hysterectomy, which removes the womb, cervix, top of the vagina and surrounding tissue. This is quite invasive, so in stage 1 vaginal cancers, it might be possible to have just radiotherapy to treat the area. In more advanced cancers, chemotherapy may also be needed.

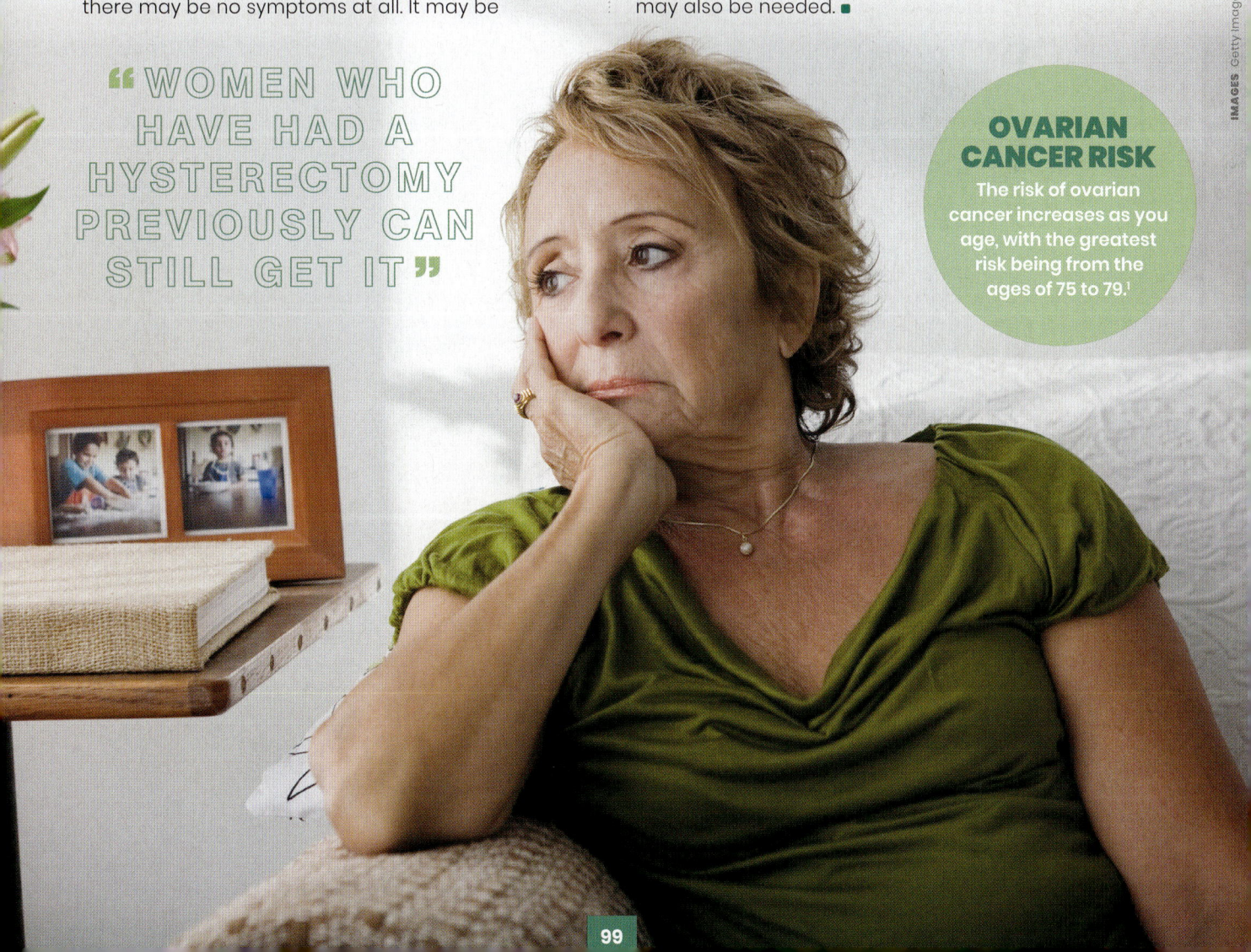

Gynaecological Cancers

SOURCES: [1] Cancer Research UK. [2] World Health Organization. IMAGES Getty Images

> "WOMEN WHO HAVE HAD A HYSTERECTOMY PREVIOUSLY CAN STILL GET IT"

OVARIAN CANCER RISK

The risk of ovarian cancer increases as you age, with the greatest risk being from the ages of 75 to 79.[1]

Bladder, Urinary & Bowel Health

UTIs ARE COMMON
More than half of women will experience a UTI at some point in their lifetime.[1]

BLADDER, URINARY &
BOWEL HEALTH

Look after your pelvic organs to keep them functioning optimally

You might not spend too much time thinking about your pelvic organs, but problems in your bladder, urinary tract and bowel can really impact on your day-to-day life. Knowing how to look after your body's organs and functions can help you prevent some of these problems, but you should also be aware of the signs and symptoms so you can treat conditions quickly.

BLADDER AND URINARY HEALTH

Your urinary system is made up of several different organs, which work together to filter blood and remove waste. Your kidneys remove the waste products from the body and retain a delicate balance between salts and water in the blood. From each kidney, a narrow tube (ureter) carries the urine down to the bladder. Your bladder sits in your pelvis and is a hollow organ designed to expand and fill up with urine temporarily. A healthy bladder can hold about 400 to 600 millilitres of urine, and it then contracts to help pass the urine through the urethra and out of the body.

Healthy urine is a pale-yellow colour, which means that your body is in balance. Having different colours of urine can indicate a problem. Darker yellow urine is a sign that you need to drink more water; a very dark brown colour could be severe dehydration or a sign of a liver problem; while a pink or red colour suggests blood in the urine. The most important things you can do to look after your bladder is to drink enough water every day and go to the toilet when you need to – don't try to hold on to it for too long or try to pass urine when you don't need to. Keeping your pelvic floor strong can help with bladder control too.

If your urinary system stops working as it should, this can lead to infections and other health problems. The most common is getting a urinary tract infection (UTI), which can impact any part of your urinary system. You can get an infected bladder (called cystitis), urethra (urethritis) or a kidney infection. Symptoms include a burning sensation when you urinate; needing to go to the toilet more often than usual, especially at night, and more urgently; blood in your urine; cloudy or dark urine; pain in your stomach; and a high temperature. Sometimes an infection can clear up on its own, especially if you keep drinking water to help flush it out. Otherwise, you may need antibiotics to get rid of it.

Another issue with urinary health is incontinence, which is when you leak urine. This is very common and nothing to be embarrassed about. There are different types of urinary incontinence, including stress incontinence, which is when you leak when you laugh, cough or jump; urgency incontinence, which is when you have an intense and urgent need to urinate, causing a leakage; overflow incontinence, which is when you can't fully empty your bladder and the excess leaks out; and total incontinence, which is when the bladder can't store urine properly at all. The most common, particularly in women, is stress incontinence, which can be caused by weak pelvic floor muscles and can be impacted by pregnancy and childbirth.

Treatment usually involves lifestyle changes to improve your urinary health, such as being a healthy weight, limiting alcohol and not smoking; doing pelvic floor exercises; and training your bladder to hold on to urine for longer. In the meantime, you may need to use absorbent pads to help catch any leakage. There are medical and ▶

> "HAVING DIFFERENT COLOURS OF URINE CAN INDICATE A PROBLEM"

Bladder, Urinary & Bowel Health

PELVIC FLOOR

The importance of your pelvic floor and how to look after it

Your pelvic floor muscles are based in your pelvis and support your pelvic organs, including your bladder, womb, vagina and bowel. These muscles need to be strong and healthy, like any muscle, to ensure good pelvic health. You use your pelvic floor when you go to the toilet, but they also help you to be stable, balance and have a strong core. Your pelvic floor muscles can weaken with age, and also due to the impact of pregnancy and childbirth. This can lead to problems such as leaking urine, constipation and pelvic organ prolapse. You can strengthen your pelvic floor through a special set of exercises. Make sure that you're sitting or lying comfortably. Then you need to engage the muscles by gently lifting and squeezing, a bit like if you are pausing a flow of urine mid-stream. Hold the squeeze for a few counts, then gently release. You should aim to do this about ten times and repeat a few times a day. Pilates can help engage the pelvic floor too, as well as strengthen the core.

▶ surgical treatments for more severe causes of urinary incontinence, which can be discussed with a doctor.

If you do notice blood in your urine, it's important to get it checked out. It may be a sign of an easily treatable infection, but in rare cases it can also be a symptom of bladder cancer. The most common cause of bladder cancer is smoking, which is estimated to account for about a third of all cases, as well as exposure to other harmful substances, but it's also more common in older adults. Kidney cancer can also present as blood in your urine, alongside a lump under your ribs or in your neck, pain, losing weight without trying, a high temperature and fatigue.

BOWEL HEALTH

As well as looking after your bladder, you must keep your bowels working effectively too. The bowel is part of the digestive system, which works to process the food we eat, extracting all the nutrients and expelling the waste products. The small bowel, also known as the small intestine, passes food through from the stomach and into the colon (also called the large bowel or large intestine). The small bowel is about two centimetres wide and very long, about six to eight metres, and as food passes through, it absorbs liquid and nutrients. The colon is shorter at about two metres, but wider – about six to seven centimetres. As well as also removing any remaining nutrients and liquid, the colon stores the waste and helps to pass it out of the body via the rectum and anus. Inside the colon is our gut microbiome, thousands of bacteria that help to process the food we eat.

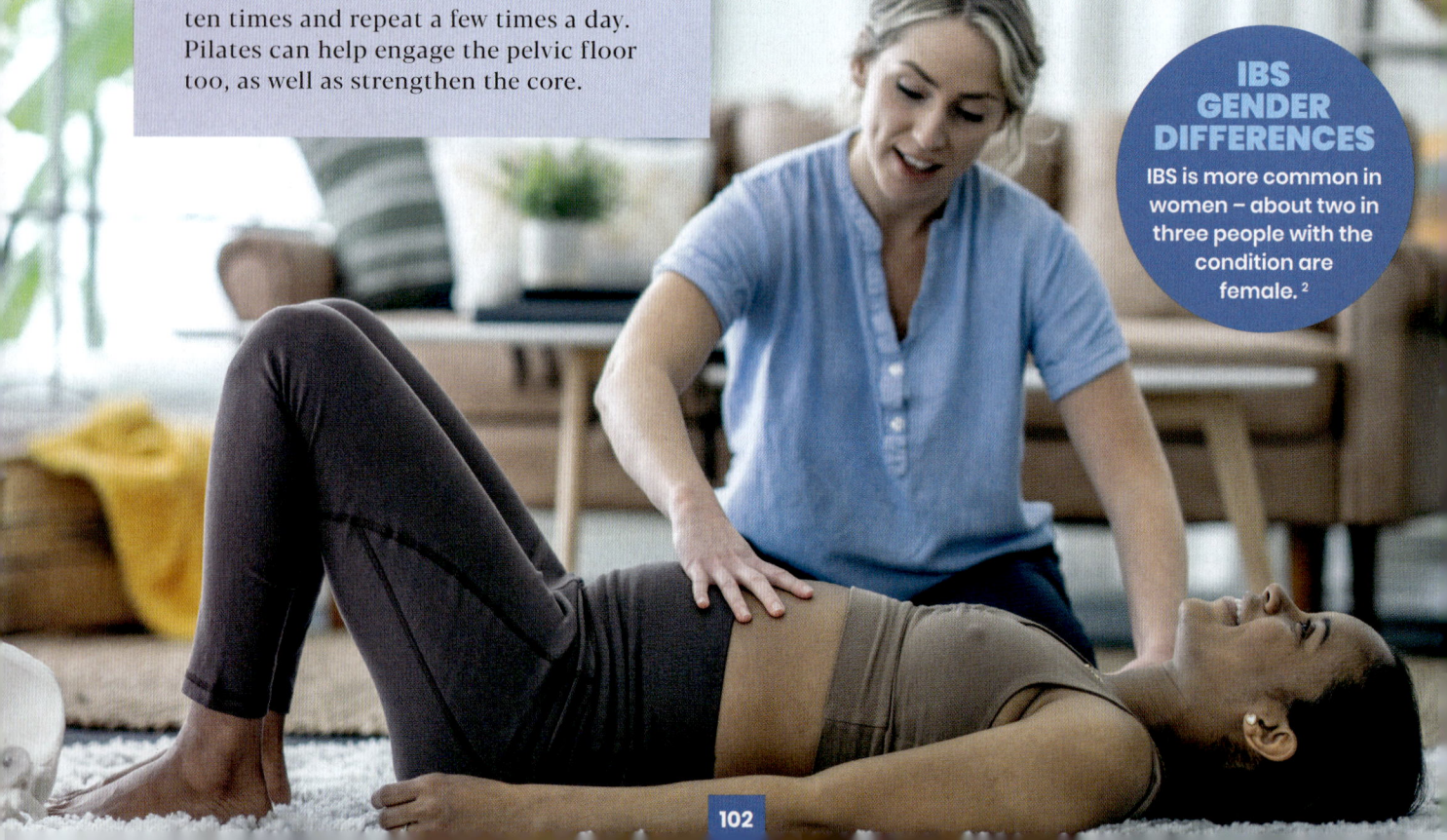

IBS GENDER DIFFERENCES
IBS is more common in women – about two in three people with the condition are female. [2]

To maintain good bowel health, you need to eat regular, healthy meals. Fibre helps to produce a healthy stool (poo) that can be easily passed out of the body, which means you need to ensure you eat enough fibrous wholegrains, fruit and vegetables, legumes and pulses, aiming for about 30 grams a day. Drinking enough water also helps to keep your bowel healthy, as does doing regular exercise.

If you don't have enough fibre, are sedentary or don't drink enough fluids, this can cause the stool to harden and move more slowly through your bowel, making it hard to pass – this is constipation. Some medications can also cause constipation, so make sure you're drinking enough water to compensate. You may need to take short-term laxatives to clear the problem, which help to soften the stool. The opposite problem is diarrhoea, which is when your stools are watery and loose. Commonly, this is due to gastroenteritis, an infection of the bowel, causing waste to move too quickly through the bowels before the fluid and nutrients can be absorbed. This could be due to a bacterial infection, a virus or a parasite, as well as other bowel conditions. Mostly this clears up on its own, but you need to ensure that you're taking plenty of fluids in to replace what you're losing.

> **"DRINKING ENOUGH WATER KEEPS YOUR BOWEL HEALTHY"**

Some people suffer from bowel conditions that affect how the bowel works. Inflammatory bowel disease (IBD) describes conditions that cause stomach pain and diarrhoea. You may also have blood in your stool, fatigue and unexpected weight loss. There are different types of IBD, but the main ones are Crohn's disease and ulcerative colitis. Crohn's disease is a chronic and lifelong condition where parts of the digestive system are inflamed; it can't be cured, but there are medicines to reduce inflammation or surgery to remove part of the bowel. It often starts in childhood or young adulthood. Ulcerative colitis is when the colon and rectum become inflamed. Symptoms can come and go, and vary in severity, but a flare-up can be very painful and distressing. Ulcerative colitis is thought to be an autoimmune condition, where the body's immune system attacks healthy tissue.

IBD is different to irritable bowel syndrome (IBS), which is a more common condition that causes stomach cramps, bloating, diarrhoea and constipation. It can't usually be cured completely, but lifestyle changes can help. This includes avoiding ultraprocessed foods and cooking with fresh ingredients, managing stress and exercising. A food diary to identify triggers might help, as can taking probiotics. ∎

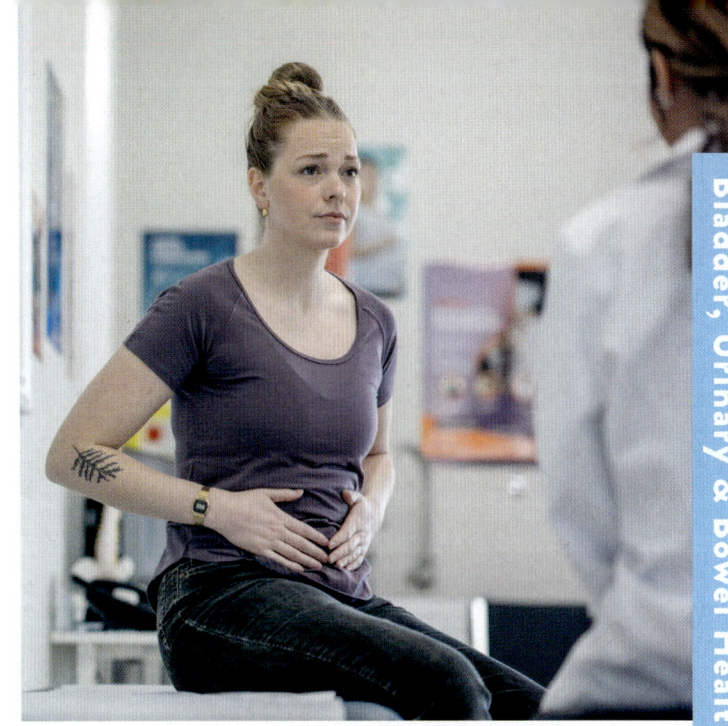

BOWEL CANCER

Early detection is so important, so know how to spot the signs and symptoms

Bowel cancer, or colorectal cancer, is the third most common cancer in the world and accounts for around 10% of all cancer cases.[3] It's when cancer is found anywhere in the large bowel, including the colon and the rectum. If detected early, it's easier to treat with a higher chance of success. Bowel cancer screening, which is advised from age 45 (USA) or 54 (UK), can help with early detection, but it's really important to be aware of the signs, as it's possible to develop bowel cancer at any age. The main symptoms include a change in your bowel habits, which could be needing to go to the toilet more or less often than usual for you; having constipation or diarrhoea that's not usual for you; bleeding from your bottom; blood in your poo; stomach pain or a lump in your stomach; fatigue; and bloating. While these symptoms can be a sign of many health conditions, it's important to get checked out to find the underlying cause.

BREAST HEALTH

Learn how to care for your breasts and spot the signs of health conditions

Everyone's breasts are different, but they are all equally important. Breasts play a vital role in reproduction, as well as in sexual function and pleasure. They will develop throughout our lifetime, responding to hormones, as well as changes to our body shape. Whatever their size or shape, they deserve to be looked after with care as part of our overall health. This means looking after the skin, protecting the fibres and ligaments through adequate support, and monitoring them for any unexpected changes.

LOOKING AFTER YOUR BREASTS

Your breasts respond to both internal and external stimuli. During your menstrual cycle, they will respond to the normal fluctuations in hormones. As oestrogen increases, the milk ducts may swell, which can make your breasts feel fuller, heavy and more lumpy than usual. Then as your oestrogen drops again, this subsides. Some women also find that their breasts become more sensitive or tender before their period. During pregnancy, the breasts undergo huge changes. Tenderness and soreness can often be one of the first signs of pregnancy, and they will continue to grow throughout the pregnancy as they prepare to lactate once the baby is born. At menopause, women often notice changes to their breasts, again because of hormones. This is all very normal and a natural response to what's happening in our body.

It's important to look after the breasts properly and keep them in good health. This means wearing the right kind of bra, in the right size, for whatever we're doing. Wearing a bra that fits correctly helps us to maintain good posture. Some women with larger breasts may struggle with back pain, but a well-fitted and supportive bra can relieve the symptoms. If you're doing intense exercise, then you will need a sports bra, which is designed to protect the breasts by limiting their movement. When you're running, for example, your breasts move up and down, side to side, and in and out, by up to about 15 centimetres. Unsupported, this can lead to straining the delicate ligaments in the breasts, causing pain and stretching the skin beyond its normal range.

You also need to look after the skin of your breasts. They go through a lot, so give your breasts some love by using moisturiser to keep your skin well hydrated and supple. Opt for a gentle and fragrance-free moisturiser as the skin is sensitive. Don't forget to apply your sunscreen, too – the skin here can burn easily, so you should always use a high enough factor across your chest where it is exposed.

> **"WEARING A BRA THAT FITS CORRECTLY HELPS US TO MAINTAIN GOOD POSTURE"**

You need to learn what's normal for your breasts. The only way you can detect when anything is wrong is if you are familiar with them. This means knowing how they normally look on both sides, whether there is any skin puckering, if you have any freckles or marks, the colour and shape of your nipples, and so on. You can do this easily in a mirror so you can really get to know what is normal for you. You need to set aside time every month to check your breasts manually too. Ideally, this should not be while you're on your period, when your breasts can feel lumpier and heavier anyway, but you should be consistent at picking the same time each month. The idea of a self-examination is to look for lumps in your chest or armpit, to find any sores or ulcers, to check for nipple discharge, to spot a change in ▶

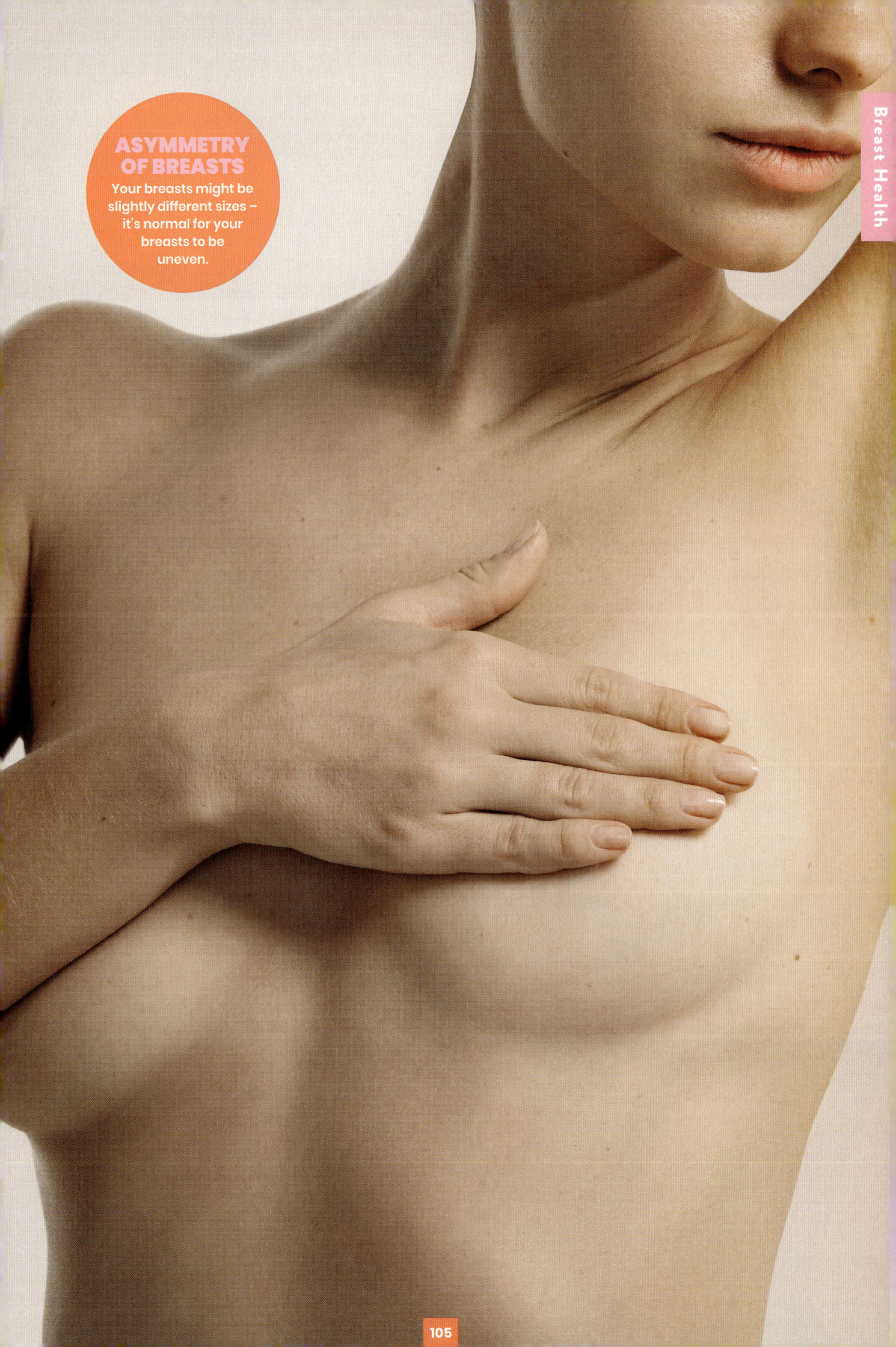

ASYMMETRY OF BREASTS
Your breasts might be slightly different sizes – it's normal for your breasts to be uneven.

Breast Health

Breast Health

AGE RISK
Most cases of breast cancer occur in women over the age of 50 and have hormonal factors.

HOW TO PERFORM A
BREAST CHECK

Examine your breasts each month to ensure they stay healthy

It's best to perform a breast check in front of a mirror, so you can see what you're doing, and to do it at the same time every month. You might want to do this lying down in bed or when you're in the shower, for example. Make sure you won't be disturbed so that you don't rush the check.

LOOK
First, stand in front of the mirror and look at your breasts. Do it first with your arms down by your side and then again with your arms in the air. You're looking for any visible changes to the skin texture, colour or appearance.

FEEL
Next you need to feel your breasts. Feel down the side of your breasts and under your armpit, checking for any swellings, lumps or hard areas. Move across the top of the breast and chest, and then feel all around the breast in a circular motion. Finally, feel under the breast and around the nipple area, not forgetting behind the nipple. Make sure that you check all the way up to your collarbones too.

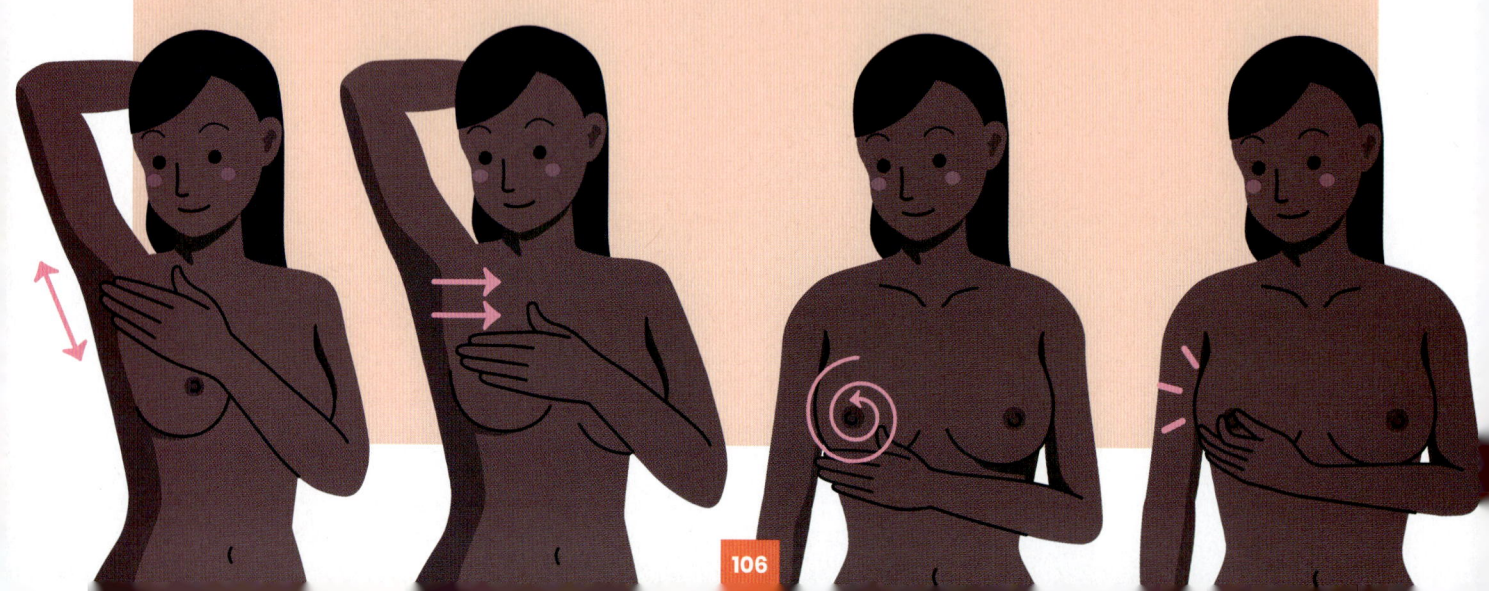

106

▸ the size of one or both breasts, or to see changes to the skin texture. We have included a how-to guide for breast checking on page 106.

COMMON BREAST PROBLEMS

There are any number of conditions that can impact on the breasts (not including breast cancer, which we will come to).

BREAST PAIN

Many women experience some kind of breast pain, which could be isolated in one breast or across both breasts. Sometimes these are linked to your cycle and can start around the time of ovulation, about two weeks before your period, and then ease off when your period starts. Other reasons for breast pain can be injury to the muscles in the shoulder, back or chest, which can radiate to the breasts; certain medications; and hormone changes related to pregnancy or menopause. Some other breast conditions can feature pain as a symptom too.

BREAST CYSTS AND FIBROADENOMAS

Finding a lump in your breast can be very worrying, but there are many other reasons why you might feel a lump or swelling. A breast cyst is a very common reason for a lump, which can feel either hard or soft, and they are usually round or oval. They can grow quickly and to any size, and they may feel painful to touch. You can have one or many cysts at the same time. Anyone can get a breast cyst, but they are more common in women over 35 and less common once you've gone through menopause. They are normally caused by the milk glands filling up with fluid and are linked to hormonal changes. They are usually diagnosed by either a mammogram or ultrasound scan, and sometimes by inserting a fine needle to see if fluid can be drawn out to confirm it's a cyst. They don't usually need any treatment, but if they're painful or large, they can sometimes be drained.

A fibroadenoma is another kind of non-cancerous lump in the breast, most common in younger women in their 20s and 30s, though they can occur at any age, even after menopause. They don't usually cause pain and feel like a smooth lump that moves easily under the skin. Diagnosis is the same as for cysts, via scans and an attempt at aspiration; if no fluid can be drawn, then a biopsy may be taken to confirm the diagnosis. Some larger fibroadenomas may need to be surgically removed.

BREAST INFECTIONS

You can get infections in your breast, which can cause you to have warm, painful skin, a rash, swelling in the breast and a high temperature. A breast infection is called mastitis and is most common in women who are breastfeeding. It is caused by a build-up of milk in the milk ducts, but it doesn't usually need any treatment. Continuing to breastfeed can be painful, but it can help to clear the infection by unclogging the milk ducts. You can also treat the breasts with a cloth soaked in warm water to help with milk flow, or a cold compress to help with breast pain. Paracetamol or ibuprofen can help to bring down a high temperature, but don't forget to drink a lot of fluids too.

Other than breastfeeding, other causes of mastitis include having a breast implant, a weakened immune system and smoking. Sometimes a breast abscess can form, which is a painful build-up of fluid because of the infection. This needs to be checked by a doctor to confirm that it's an abscess, and may require hospital treatment. The fluid will be drained under local anaesthetic using either a needle or a small cut in the skin. It should then heal within a few days or weeks.

BREAST CANCER

Breast cancer is the most common type of cancer in women, so it's important to know what to look out for. Anyone can get breast cancer and early detection is key. Primary breast cancer – where it is localised to the breast and armpit – can be treated with curative intent. However, if it is left, it may spread beyond the breast and to other ▸

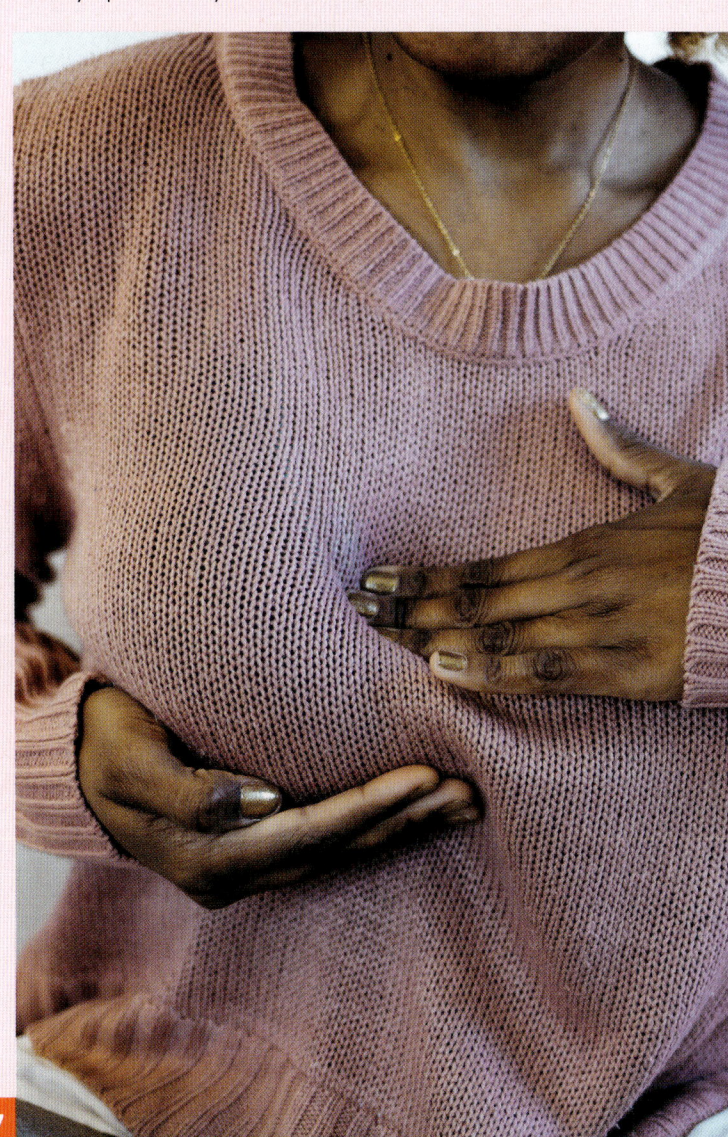

Breast Health

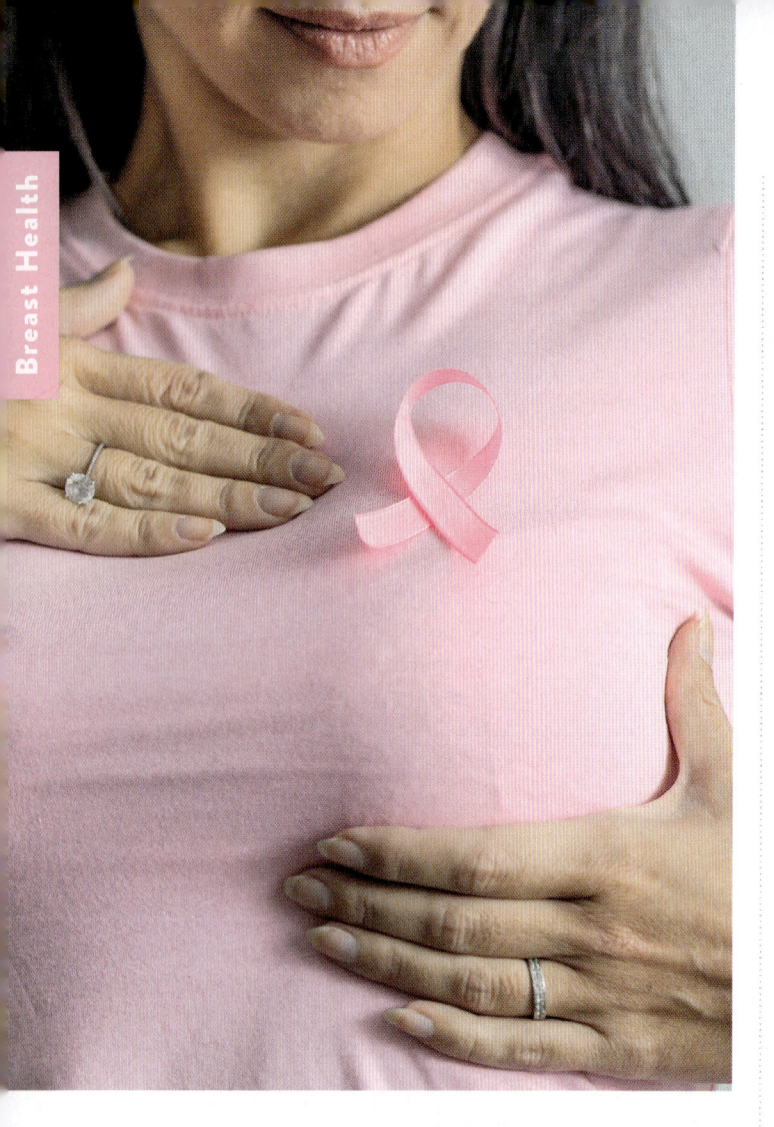

▸ parts of the body, which is called secondary breast cancer.

The main symptoms are a lump or swelling in the breast; a change in skin texture, such as dimpling or redness; a change in the shape or size of one or both breasts; nipple discharge (not linked to pregnancy or breastfeeding); changes in your nipple, such as a rash or inversion; and pain that doesn't go away. You may not get all these symptoms, which is why it's important to check your breasts regularly. Sometimes a lump is too small or too deep to be felt, so other signs can be key to getting a scan and diagnosis. If the cancer spreads, it can affect other organs such as the bones, liver, lungs or brain, which can have different symptoms.

There are different types of breast cancer, which can impact how it's treated. A cancer can either be invasive or non-invasive, which determines whether it has the ability to spread beyond the breast. Ductal carcinoma in situ (DCIS) is a very early type of non-invasive breast cancer, which is when cancer cells are detected within the milk ducts and haven't spread into the surrounding breast tissue. Caught at this stage, DCIS can be treated before the cells develop further and become invasive, though it is more difficult to catch early as it may cause no symptoms.

Most breast cancers are invasive, which means they have the potential to spread to other parts of the body. Most women with breast cancer will have invasive ductal breast cancer, which means the cancer has started and spread from the ducts. Sometimes the cancer is invasive lobular breast cancer, which is when the cancer has started and spread from the lobules. Inflammatory breast cancer is rarer and grows fast, causing skin to be red and inflamed, and caused by breast cancer cells blocking the lymph channels in the breast.

Breast cancer is treated with a combination of surgery – either to remove the lump (lumpectomy or wide local excision) but preserve the breast; or fully remove the breast (mastectomy) – chemotherapy and radiotherapy. Not every cancer will need all three treatments, as it depends on how fast the cancer is growing, how big it is, its type and whether it has spread.

Some breast cancers are driven by hormones, so when a biopsy is taken it is checked for hormone receptors, which can help the cancer to grow. Cancer cells are also tested for HER2, a protein involved in the growth of cancer cells. Cancers are categorised as to whether they are positive or negative for oestrogen receptors, progesterone receptors and HER2. Around 70-80% of breast cancers are positive for oestrogen receptors (ER+). Most breast cancers that are progesterone receptor positive (PR+) are also ER+; very rarely are cancers ER- and PR+. All hormone-positive cancers are usually treated with hormone therapy, which helps to block or lower the amount of hormones in the body.

> "SOME BREAST CANCERS ARE DRIVEN BY HORMONES"

Some breast cancers are also HER2-positive, which means they have higher-than-normal levels of this protein. This is found in fewer than one in five invasive breast cancers, and there are targeted treatments for this. If a cancer is ER+, PR+ and HER2+, this is called triple positive breast cancer. However, if the cancer is negative for all these tests, that is called triple negative breast cancer. Only around 15% of breast cancers are triple negative, but it seems to impact pre-menopausal women under 40 and Black women more often. It is harder to treat as there are no targeted treatments (hormone treatment would be ineffective, as there are no hormone receptors), but surgery, chemotherapy and radiotherapy can be effective.

Some women who develop breast cancer have a faulty BRCA gene, which is inherited. You may be offered genetic testing to test for this gene if you have triple negative breast cancer or a strong family history. However, most cases of breast cancer are not genetic. Age is the biggest risk factor, but having dense breast tissue and having previously had DCIS can also increase your risk, along with lifestyle factors.

Looking after your breasts, getting to know them, doing your self-examinations and seeing a doctor quickly if you are concerned are the best ways to catch breast cancer early and to ensure you receive treatment. Most referrals to a breast clinic find another benign reason for your symptoms, so try not to worry about the worst-case scenario unless you have to. ■

WHAT HAPPENS AT A MAMMOGRAM

It can be scary the first time you have your breasts scanned – here's what to expect

Whether you've been called up for routine breast screening, or you've been referred by a doctor, you will likely have a mammogram (and sometimes an ultrasound as well). A mammogram consists of four x-rays, two on each breast. These are performed by a specialist mammographer who ensures that you get clear scans so they can be read by an expert to spot any problem areas. You will need to undress from the waist up to perform the exam. The mammographer will then help you get in the right position on the scanning machine – you will be standing, with one breast placed on a plate, and your arm stretched out to one side. When the scan starts, your breast will be squeezed between two plates to keep it still while the scan is taken. This is done on both sides of each breast. It is a quick process, but it can be uncomfortable. You won't get the results straight away and you can leave after the scan, unless you have other appointments (such as with a consultant or breast nurse, if you've been referred due to symptoms).

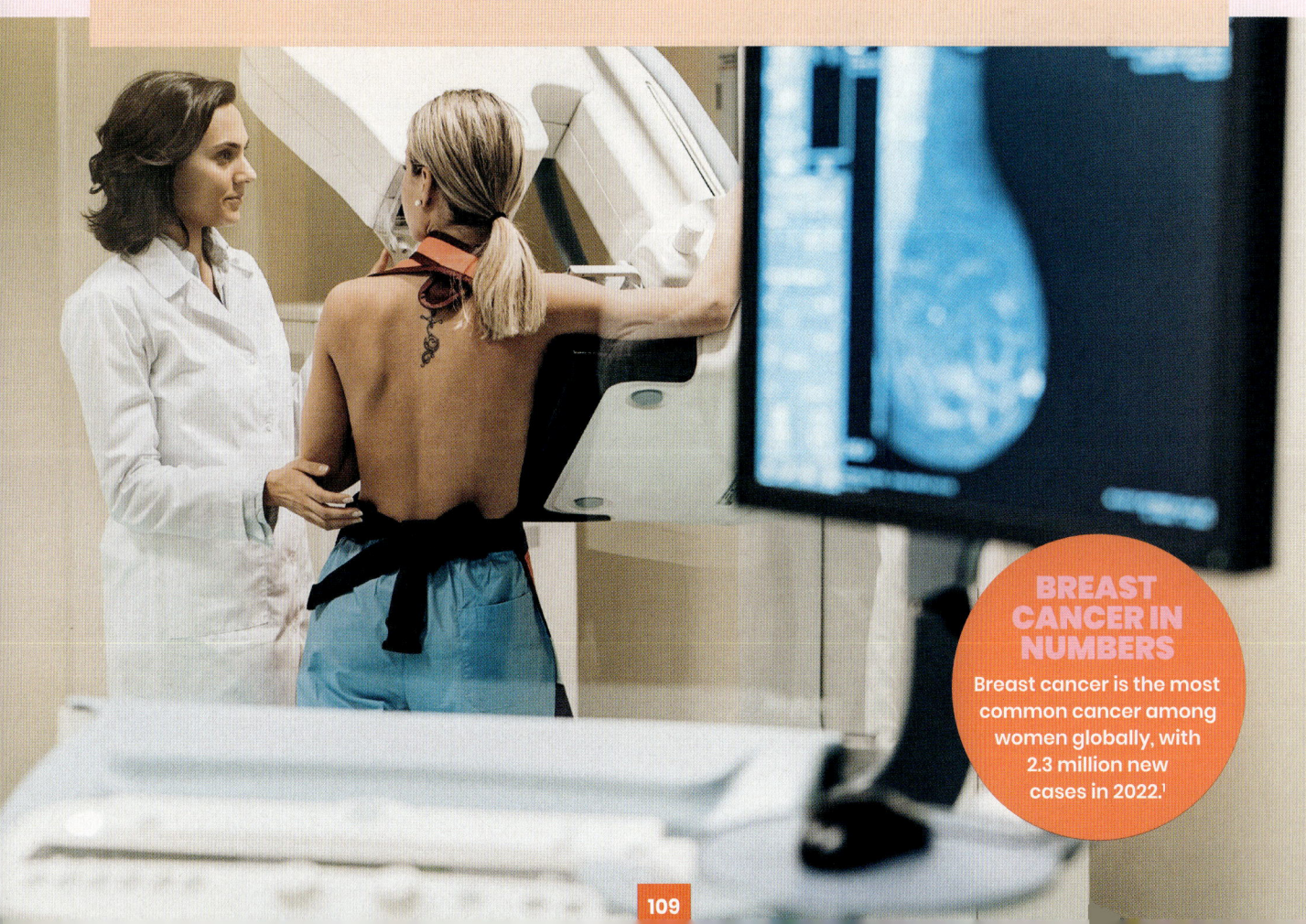

BREAST CANCER IN NUMBERS

Breast cancer is the most common cancer among women globally, with 2.3 million new cases in 2022.[1]

COMMON PROCEDURES

We explain some common medical interventions that women might undergo

HYSTERECTOMY

A hysterectomy is a procedure that removes the womb to treat various health conditions, such as very heavy periods, pelvic pain, fibroids or cancer. It is usually only considered when other options have been attempted first, as it is an invasive and major operation, with a longer recovery time. However, it is a commonly performed procedure in women and can offer long-term relief or treatment.

There are different types of hysterectomy, depending on whether other parts of your reproductive system are removed at the same time. A hysterectomy means that you won't have periods anymore and will no longer be able to carry a baby. A total hysterectomy is the most common, which removes the womb and the cervix, but leaves the ovaries and fallopian tubes intact. A radical hysterectomy is the most extreme, which removes the womb, fallopian tubes, ovaries, lymph glands, fatty tissue and part of the vagina. A subtotal hysterectomy removes the womb, but not the cervix. A total hysterectomy can also be performed alongside the removal of the ovaries (oophorectomy) and the fallopian tubes (salpingectomy).

A hysterectomy can be performed with keyhole surgery (laparoscopy) using small cuts in the stomach to remove the womb under general anaesthetic. Sometimes the womb is removed through an incision in the lower abdomen (abdominal hysterectomy), or through a cut at the top of the vagina (vaginal hysterectomy). However it is performed, there is a significant recovery period. It's possible you'll need to stay in hospital for up to five days after the operation, and then another six to eight weeks of recovery at home. If your ovaries have been removed, then you will go into menopause (a surgical menopause), and even if the ovaries are left intact, it can cause an earlier-than-normal menopause. If the cervix is removed, you will no longer need to go for cervical screening tests.

HYSTERECTOMY PREVALENCE
A hysterectomy is the second most commonly performed surgical procedure in women after a C-section.

COLPOSCOPY

This test is done to take a closer look at your cervix. A speculum is placed in the vagina to help open it up – this is the same tool used in a cervical screening. It's a plastic tube that hinges open when in place to gently widen the vagina to help the doctor see better. A microscope is then used (externally) to examine the cervix. If needed, a small sample of cells are taken to be tested. There are many reasons why a colposcopy is performed, but the most common is if you have an abnormal result from a routine cervical screening test, high-risk HPV is detected, or if the results from the cervical screening were not clear. You may also be offered a colposcopy to investigate unusual bleeding. You should ensure that you're not on your period for the examination, and you shouldn't have penetrative sex or use any period products or creams inside your vagina for 24 hours before to ensure that the cervix is clear. It's a quick procedure that only takes 15 to 20 minutes, though it may feel a little uncomfortable. Afterwards you may find that you have a little bleeding, but this should clear up quickly.

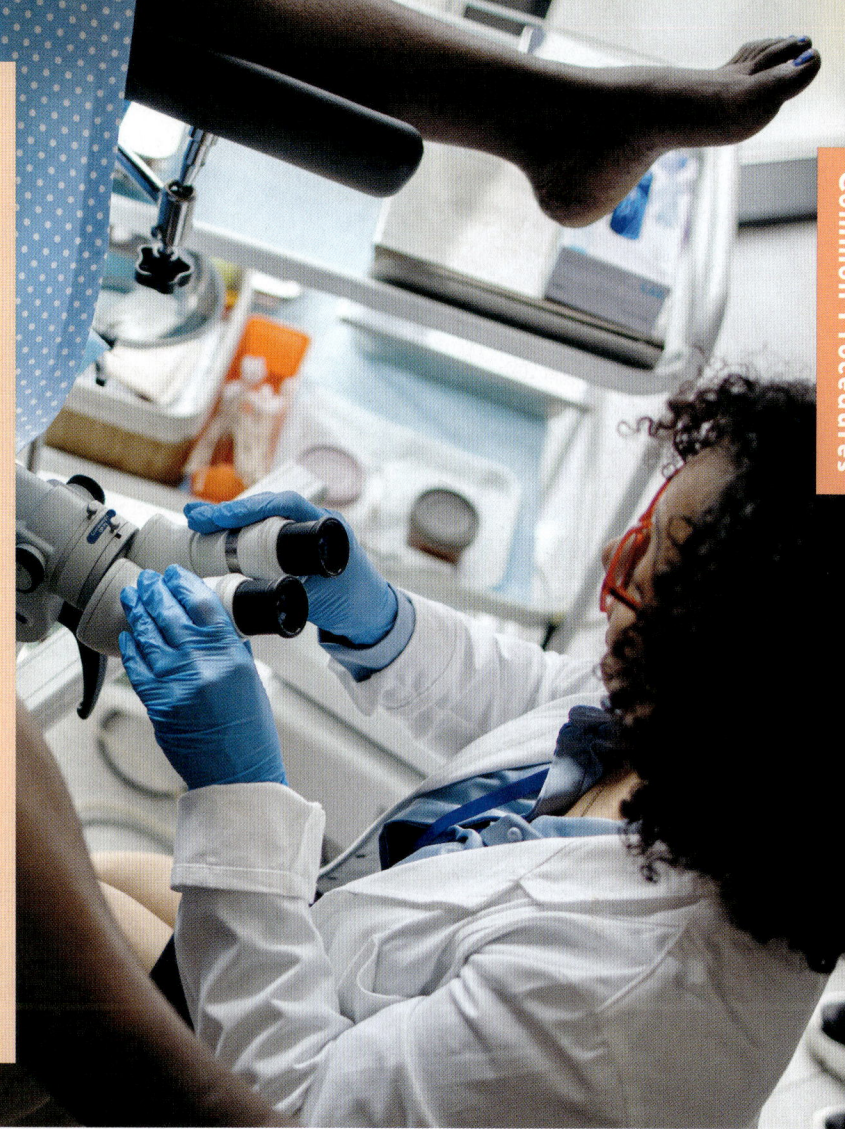

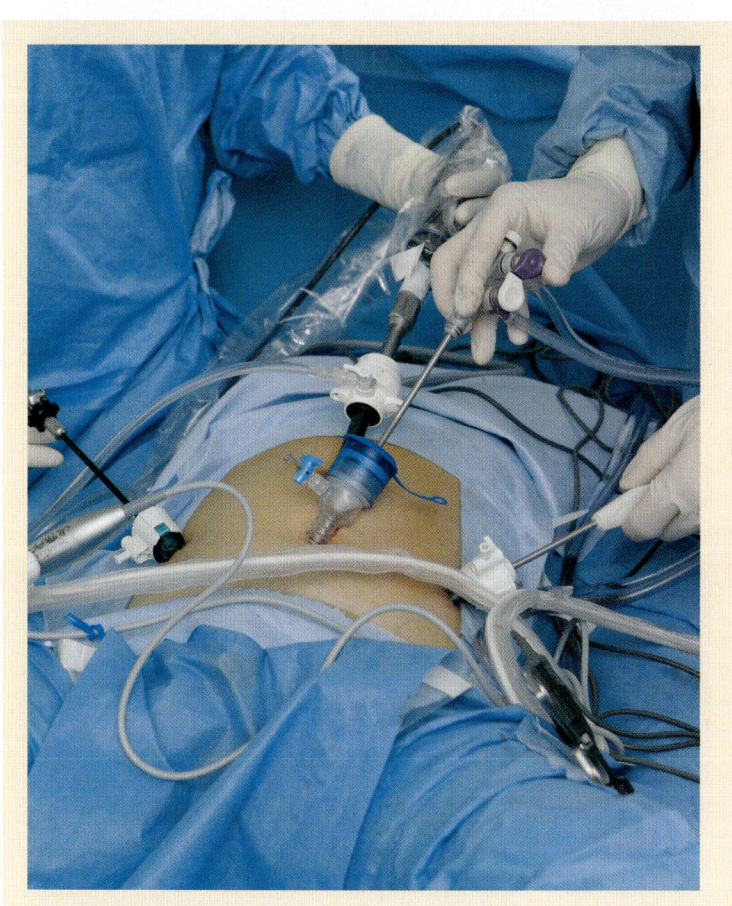

Common Procedures

MYOMECTOMY

Myomectomy is the medical term for a procedure to remove fibroids. These are non-cancerous growths in the womb that can be any size. They don't always cause symptoms, but if they do, and medicine isn't helping to relieve the symptoms, you may need to have them removed, especially if they are impacting your day-to-day life. Some women will have a hysterectomy (see the previous page), to remove the womb and the fibroids along with it, but if you are hoping to have future children, a myomectomy to remove just the fibroids may be an alternative. It is not a suitable procedure for all types of fibroids, as it depends on the size, how many there are and the position of the fibroids. A myomectomy is performed under general anaesthetic, and will either be done via keyhole surgery (numerous small cuts through your abdomen) or an open surgery (one large cut). You will likely need to recover in hospital for a couple of days, before going home to rest. It can take a few weeks to recover fully. ▶

Common Procedures

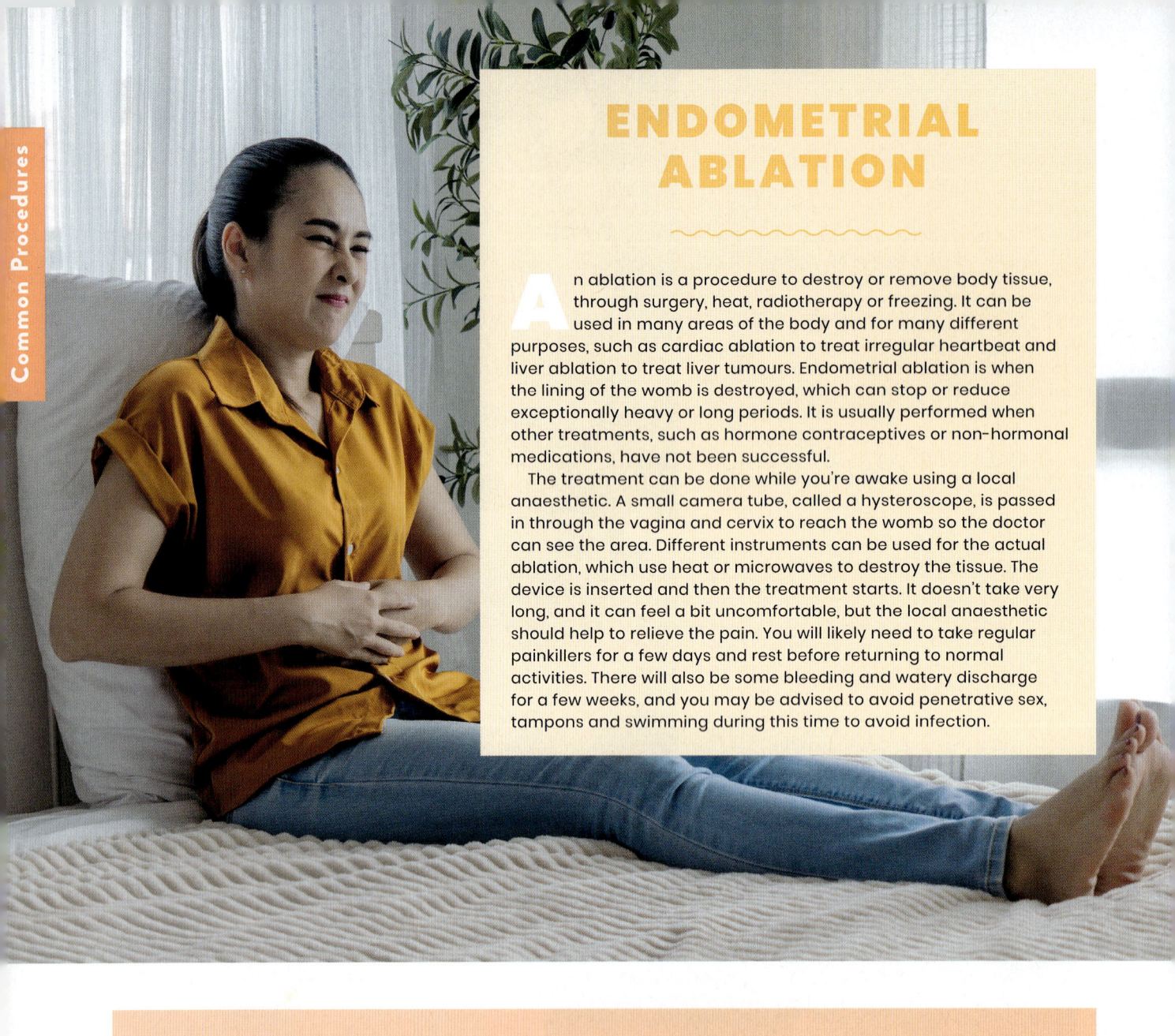

ENDOMETRIAL ABLATION

An ablation is a procedure to destroy or remove body tissue, through surgery, heat, radiotherapy or freezing. It can be used in many areas of the body and for many different purposes, such as cardiac ablation to treat irregular heartbeat and liver ablation to treat liver tumours. Endometrial ablation is when the lining of the womb is destroyed, which can stop or reduce exceptionally heavy or long periods. It is usually performed when other treatments, such as hormone contraceptives or non-hormonal medications, have not been successful.

The treatment can be done while you're awake using a local anaesthetic. A small camera tube, called a hysteroscope, is passed in through the vagina and cervix to reach the womb so the doctor can see the area. Different instruments can be used for the actual ablation, which use heat or microwaves to destroy the tissue. The device is inserted and then the treatment starts. It doesn't take very long, and it can feel a bit uncomfortable, but the local anaesthetic should help to relieve the pain. You will likely need to take regular painkillers for a few days and rest before returning to normal activities. There will also be some bleeding and watery discharge for a few weeks, and you may be advised to avoid penetrative sex, tampons and swimming during this time to avoid infection.

REMOVAL OF OVARIAN CYSTS

Both a laparoscopy and laparotomy are procedures used to remove cysts from your ovaries. These are common fluid-filled sacs that develop on an ovary, and you may not even know you have them. They are common and they often go away on their own. However, if they get too big or rupture, they can start to cause problems and impact on your daily activity. If it's decided that surgery is the best option to remove the cyst, then you will have one of two procedures. Most commonly, a laparoscopy will be performed under general anaesthetic. This is keyhole surgery when a number of small cuts are made through your stomach. Gas is then pushed into the pelvis, making it possible to access the ovaries. Using a small microscope with a light on the end (a laparoscope), a surgeon can see where the cyst is and remove it. The cut is closed with stitches that will naturally dissolve over time. If it's not possible to remove the cyst through a laparoscopy, then a laparotomy is performed instead. It's a similar operation, but open surgery with one large incision. This is sometimes done if the ovary and the cyst both need to be removed, or if there is a chance it could be cancer, to ensure the whole area is removed for testing. You will need to stay in hospital for a couple of days after this bigger operation. It can take a few months to recover from these surgeries completely.

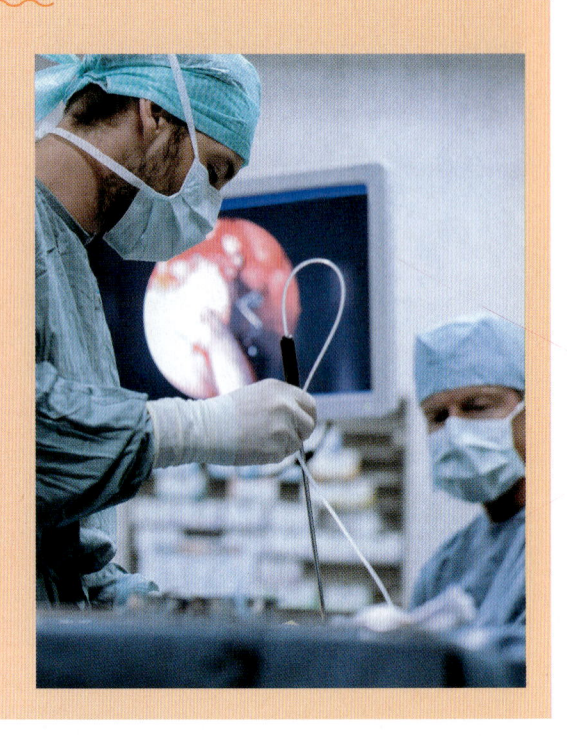

HYSTEROSCOPY

This is when a thin tube with a camera on the end is inserted into the womb through the vagina and the cervix. Salt water is injected into the womb to make it easier to see. It is used to help diagnose a range of conditions, such as fibroids or polyps (small growths), and to help find out why you might be having heavy bleeding, bleeding after menopause or problems getting pregnant. The procedure can be uncomfortable and make you feel faint or sick. It's a good idea to have some pain relief in advance; usually over-the-counter painkillers will be enough, but for some women, it can be very painful, so there may be other options. It is possible in some cases to do the procedure under sedation or general anaesthetic. Some small growths or fibroids can be removed at the same time if needed, or a biopsy taken. Afterwards, you may have some pain, similar to period-related cramps, and a bit of spotting. You should not have this procedure if there is a chance you could be pregnant.

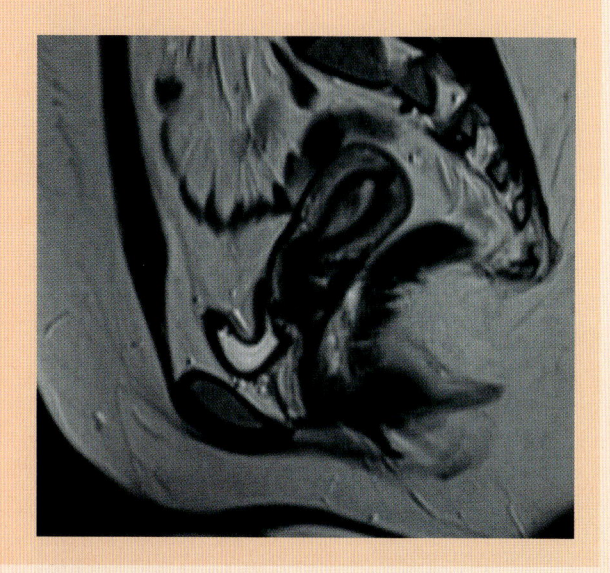

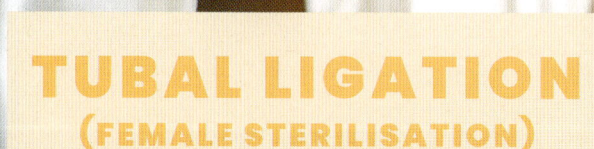

TUBAL LIGATION
(FEMALE STERILISATION)

You might hear this procedure referred to as 'having your tubes tied', as it involves blocking off your fallopian tubes. It's an efficient form of contraception – 99% effective at preventing pregnancy. While it can sometimes be reversed, that's not always possible or available. Therefore, it's important to ensure that you don't want to have any, or any more, children. Other contraception options may be offered, or you may want to discuss your options with a doctor, nurse or counsellor before deciding.

The operation is performed under a general anaesthetic and takes 20 to 30 minutes. Small cuts are made through your abdomen, and gas is pumped in to make it easier to see your organs. A small camera is passed through to help the surgeon see your fallopian tubes. Your fallopian tubes will then be sealed, blocked or partially removed, before the cut is closed with dissolvable stitches. It's normally a day procedure, and you may have some light bleeding and pain for a few days afterwards. You can usually stop using your normal contraception about seven days after the operation. You will continue to have periods, and your hormone levels should be unaffected.

RECOVERY
It's important to listen to advice on rest and recovery after any procedure to ensure that you do heal properly.

HEALTH SCREENINGS

Screenings are essential for catching problems as early as possible – they could save your life

GET IT DONE!
It can feel embarrassing or uncomfortable, but these screenings are essential for early detection and peace of mind.

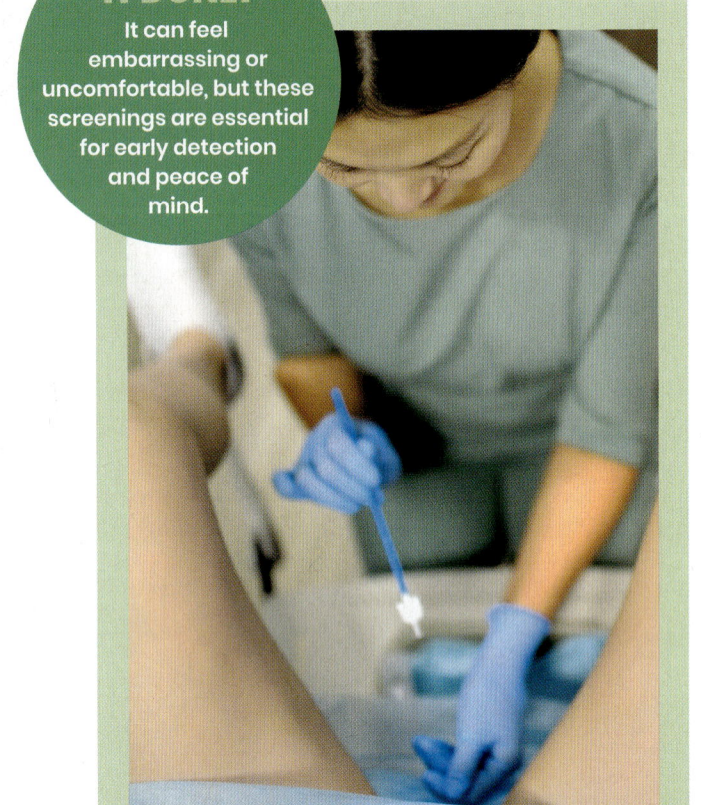

CERVICAL SCREENING

All women should be having routine cervical screening tests. These are sometimes also known as Pap tests or smear tests. During a screening, a small sample of cells is taken from the cervix and then analysed to look for certain types of human papillomavirus (HPV). HPV can cause changes to the cells in the cervix, which then have the potential to develop into cancer. By catching the HPV early enough, it's possible to treat before it develops or causes these cell changes. An HPV vaccine is offered to girls and boys at around the age of 12 to 13 years to offer protection against HPV.

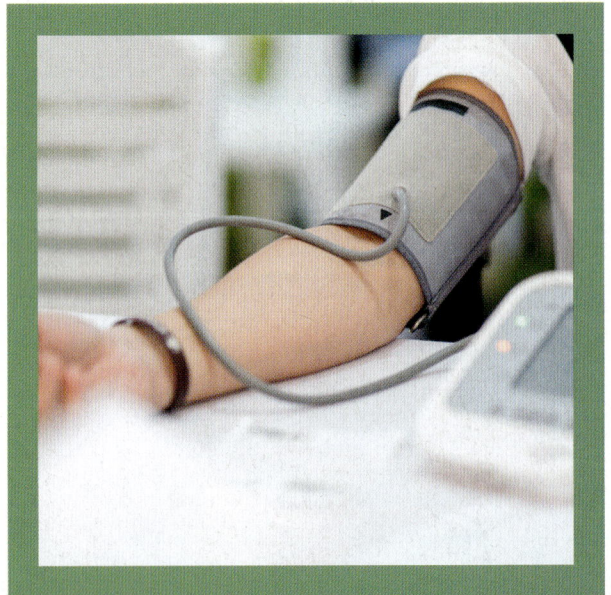

BLOOD PRESSURE CHECKS

There are rarely any signs of high blood pressure, unless it gets particularly high, so the only way to know if you have high blood pressure is to get it checked. You can get home blood pressure devices, but it is still worth getting blood pressure checked properly as home machines can have a margin of error. You can get your blood pressure checked at your doctor's surgery or a pharmacy. Some workplaces also offer routine blood pressure checks. In the UK, there is also an NHS Health Check offered to people over 40, which includes blood pressure tests, along with cholesterol checks and other measures of good health.

> **THERE ARE RARELY ANY SIGNS OF HIGH BLOOD PRESSURE, SO GET IT CHECKED**

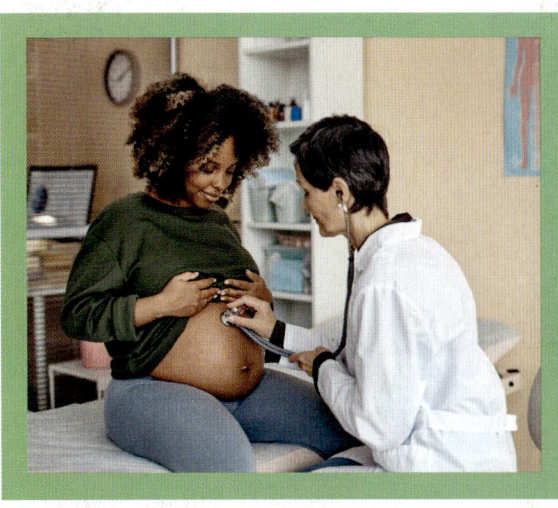

SCREENINGS IN PREGNANCY

During pregnancy, you will have regular check-ups for both you and the baby. When it comes to monitoring your health, screenings offered include checking for infectious diseases like hepatitis B or HIV. Checks can also be done for certain inheritable conditions, like sickle cell disease. Women at a higher risk of developing diabetes during pregnancy will also have their glucose levels checked. Throughout pregnancy, samples will be taken to monitor for signs of pre-eclampsia. We cover more on screenings for mother and baby in our section on pregnancy.

DIABETIC EYE SCREENING

If you are diabetic, then you will have annual check-ups to ensure that you're managing your condition. One important test that also needs to be done regularly is an eye test looking for signs of diabetic retinopathy, which is triggered by high blood-sugar levels damaging the retina. If it's not caught, it can cause sight problems and even sight loss. The screening can detect changes early, which means that the condition can be treated, often before you even notice a problem with your eyes.

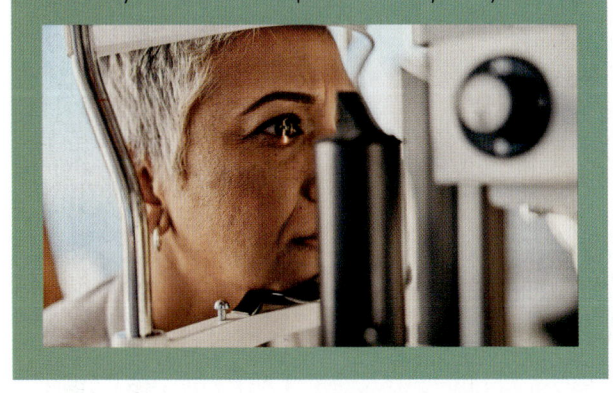

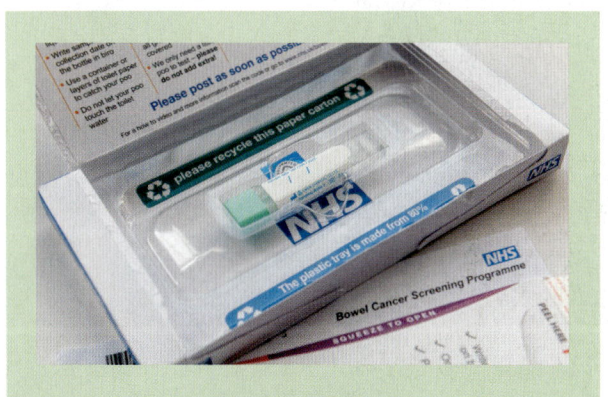

BOWEL SCREENING

Bowel screening can usually be done at home, and involves having to provide a stool (poo) sample using a home kit that is then analysed to check for any signs of bowel cancer. In the UK, bowel screening is offered to everyone aged 54 to 74, but the age is lowering to 50. In the USA, it's recommended to start screenings from the age of 45. The screening can detect tiny amounts of blood in faeces, which can be a sign of bowel cancer and is one of the best ways of detecting it early.

BREAST SCREENING

Women should start having routine mammograms – breast screenings – from the age of 50. However, if there is a family history of breast cancer or other underlying reasons, you may be advised to start screenings from a younger age. Screenings should then be done at least every three years, unless advised otherwise, and as long as the previous screening detected no problems. During a mammogram, your breasts are scanned by a special type of x-ray machine by placing them one at a time between two plates. This can be a bit uncomfortable, but it doesn't take long. The scans can then be analysed to detect the early signs of breast cancer.

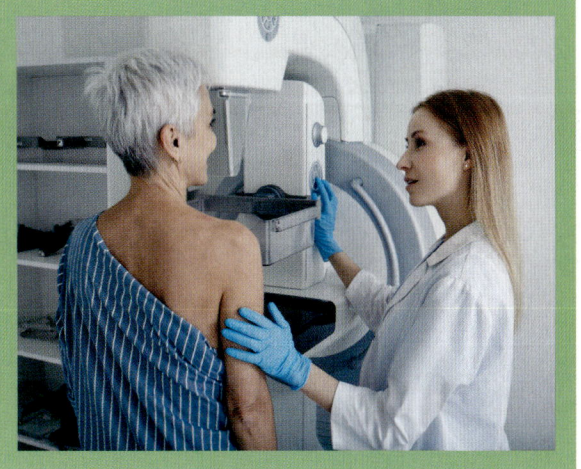

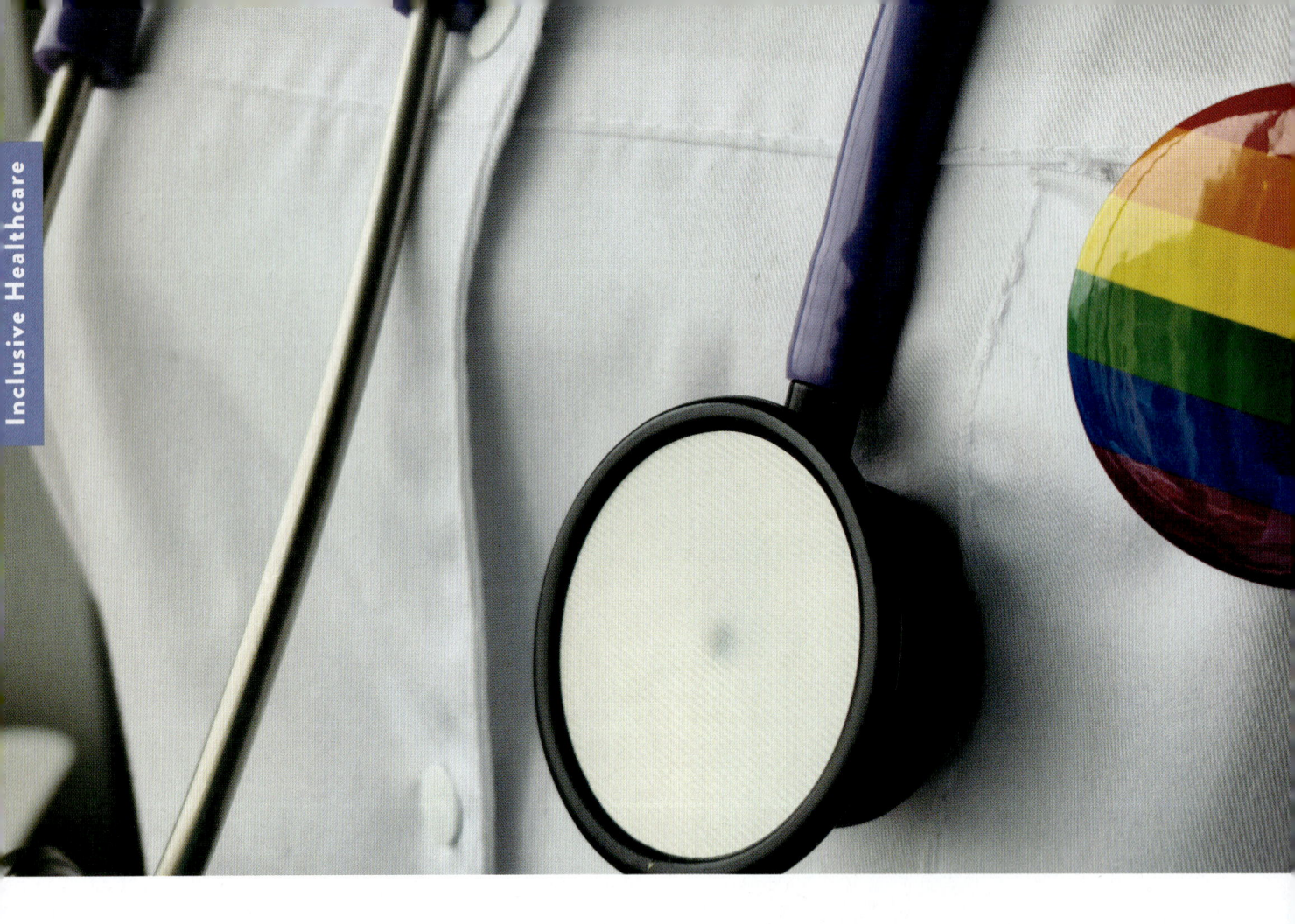

INCLUSIVE HEALTHCARE

Anyone with a cervix, womb or other reproductive organs needs to be aware of screening tests and symptoms of health conditions

It's important for transgender, non-binary and intersex people to be aware of conditions that might impact their health, even if their gender identity is different to their assigned sex at birth. It can be distressing and difficult to consider gynaecological health and there is a lack of information and advice, which can make it hard to know what to do if you develop concerns or if you are having unusual symptoms.

If you have had any type of surgery or hormonal interventions, this might impact on certain aspects of your health, and the signs, symptoms and risks of certain health conditions may be different. This is why it's so important to know what is normal for your body so you can be aware of any changes.

IMPORTANT CHECKS

If you have a womb, cervix, ovaries, fallopian tubes, vagina or vulva, then there is a risk of the main gynaecological cancers. We have a section in this book dedicated to the five main cancers, along with their signs and symptoms, so it is useful to be aware of these. If you have breast tissue, then there

GET SUPPORT
It's important to have someone to talk to – whether a friend, family member or support group.

RESOURCES FOR TRANS & NON-BINARY PEOPLE

If you need more advice and support regarding health concerns, here are some online resources

THE EVE APPEAL
eveappeal.org.uk
The Eve Appeal is a gynaecological cancer charity that has advice and information for transgender, non-binary and intersex people, as well as good-practice tips for healthcare professionals.

TRANSACTUAL
transactual.org.uk
Here you can find a lot of information on trans-inclusive healthcare, including getting support from your doctor, mental health and common issues. It also has a detailed list of other trans-inclusive services.

QUEER MENOPAUSE
queermenopause.com
Advice and information for anyone experiencing menopause, with lots of support and resources to answer common questions and concerns.

TERRENCE HIGGINS TRUST
tht.org.uk
This charity website has advice on sexual health for transgender and non-binary people.

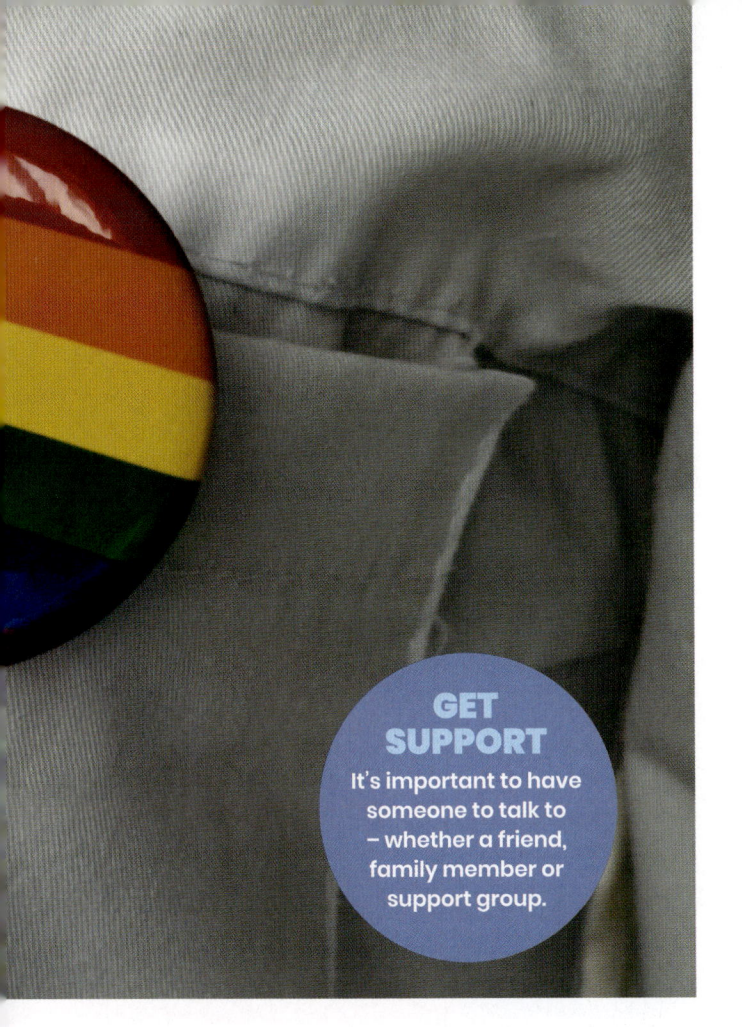

is a risk of breast cancer, and again we have information in this book about breast care, self-checks and symptoms of breast cancer. You may feel uncomfortable when it comes to performing these self-examinations, but early detection of problems can mean that treatment is much more successful.

You also need to be aware of the screenings that are available to you and your options around them. This includes things like cervical screenings and mammograms, which are important checks that can catch early cases of cancer. In the UK, trans men and non-binary people who were both assigned female at birth, and are registered with a doctor as female, will continue to be invited for breast and cervical screenings as per the usual schedule. Trans men and non-binary people who were assigned female at birth and are registered with a doctor as male will not be routinely invited for breast and cervical screenings, though you have the right to request them.

In other countries around the world, access to healthcare is different and you would need to check what is usual in your region. It is recommended that you have a routine breast screening if you have not had chest reconstruction or if you still have breast tissue. It is also recommended that you have routine cervical screening if you have a cervix.

Going for a screening can be an upsetting experience, as it involves intimate checks in a clinical environment. You can speak to the doctor or nurse before the appointment to explain your concerns. You may be able to request that your appointment is made at the beginning or end of the day, for example, so that you don't have to be in the waiting room among other people, and to ensure more privacy.

Peer support groups can be useful to help talk through feelings around self-examination and going for screenings. You could also ask a trusted person to accompany you to appointments to help advocate for your needs. Your health is important, so it's better to ask for adjustments to ensure you can access healthcare, than it is not to access services at all.

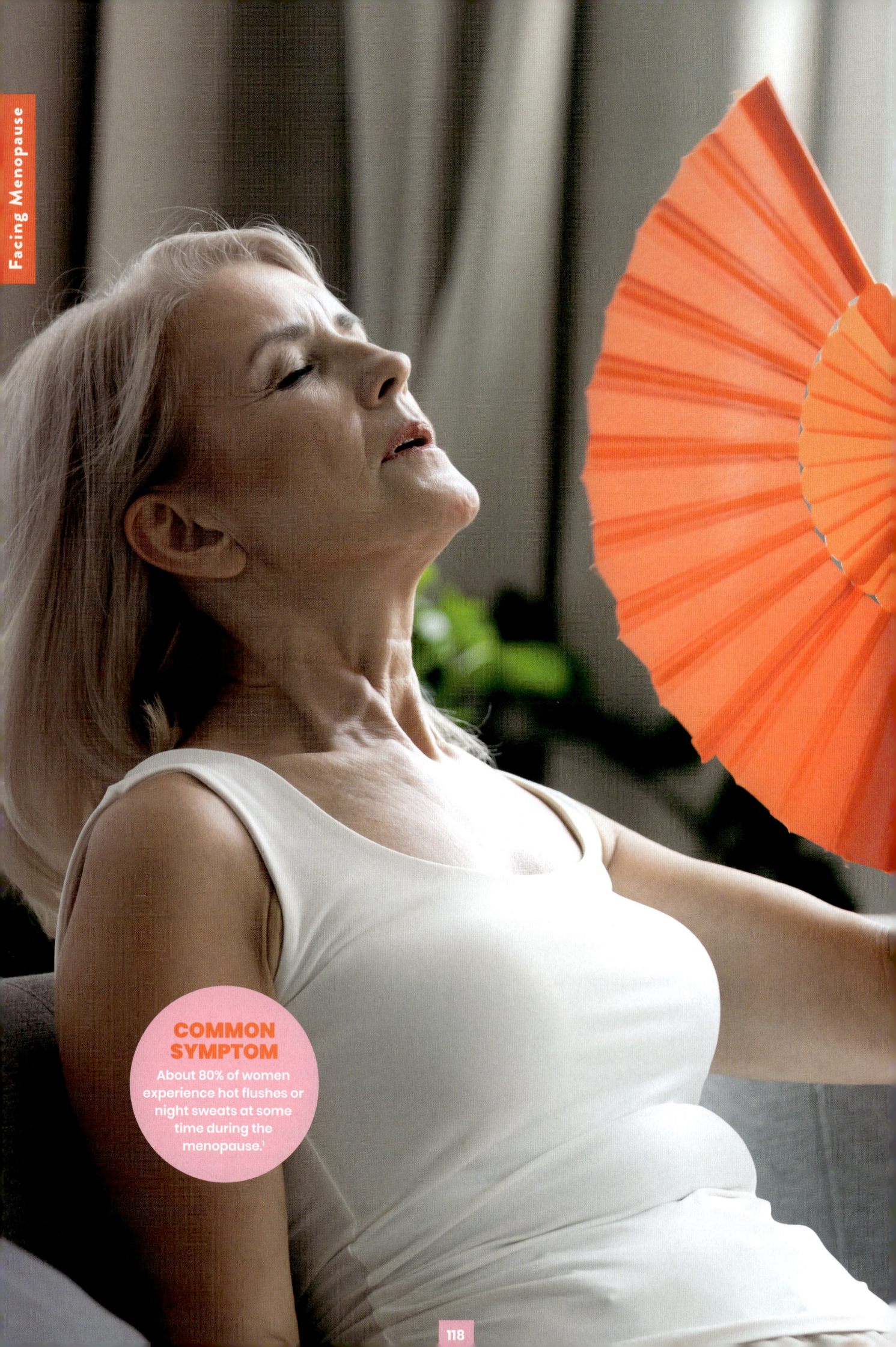

Facing Menopause

COMMON SYMPTOM
About 80% of women experience hot flushes or night sweats at some time during the menopause.[1]

FACING MENOPAUSE

Menopause is a natural stage in a woman's life, like puberty, and it comes with its challenges

Menopause is a time of big hormonal changes, causing symptoms that can affect your physical and mental health. It can be overwhelming thinking about this phase and the changes it will bring, but it doesn't have to be a negative experience. With the right lifestyle choices, and access to appropriate treatment and symptom relief, menopause can be a manageable, even positive, time of life.

WHAT IS MENOPAUSE?

The path to menopause begins before we're even born. When a foetus grows in the womb, ovaries are one of the earliest organs to develop. At 20 weeks, the foetus will have a fully developed reproductive system with many millions of eggs. This will be a woman's entire lifetime supply of eggs, and they start to decline in number immediately. At birth, a female baby will have around one to two million eggs. Throughout childhood, this number keeps going down, and you'll likely have 300,000 to 500,000 eggs by the time you have your first period.

Every cycle, multiple eggs begin the process of ovulation, but only one follicle will mature and release an egg, while the rest of the eggs will be reabsorbed by the body. As you age, your ovaries will begin to atrophy, decreasing the number and quality of your remaining eggs. In turn, this slows down the production of hormones. At first, your hormone levels might rise and fall, which is what can cause the symptoms associated with menopause. You're still fertile at this point as long as you're having periods, even if they're not as regular as they used to be.

Eventually, your periods will slow down and then stop altogether. This doesn't mean that you've run out of eggs – even at menopause, a woman can still have around 1,000 eggs remaining, but they are no longer viable. The timescale at which this happens is different from woman to woman. Some women might have a few symptoms and their periods stop within a few months; whereas others will have symptoms for up to ten years before they reach the point of menopause. You'll never really know when your period is your last period, as there can be a long gap between cycles, which is why menopause is determined to be a year after your last period, because at this point it's unlikely you'll have another one. On average, the time between your hormone levels starting to drop and your last period is around seven years.

> **"THE AVERAGE AGE OF MENOPAUSE IS 51 YEARS OLD, ALTHOUGH THIS CAN VARY A LOT"**

STAGES OF MENOPAUSE

There are three stages of menopause, though we tend to use it as an umbrella term for the whole process, encompassing all three stages.

Menopause itself means the end of your monthly cycles. It is when you have your last-ever period, so it is in fact just a single day, from which point on you will never have a period again. The average age of menopause is 51 years old, but this can vary a lot. Some women go through an earlier-than-usual menopause (see the box on the next page), but anything between 45 to 55 years old is normal.

The most significant stage of menopause, and the one that's talked about most often due to the symptoms associated with it, is perimenopause (or pre-menopause). This is the time in which you transition from your reproductive years into menopause. This stage normally begins some time in your 40s, with an average age of 46 to 47 years old. Some women will start having symptoms in ▸

their late 30s. It's when your hormone levels are at their most erratic and uncontrollable, but not everyone has a hard time with perimenopause.

There is no definite way to diagnose perimenopause. There are hormone tests that can be done, for example, to check your FSH and LH levels, but these naturally fluctuate from hour to hour and day to day, so a test taken on one day can't determine for certain if you're heading towards menopause. Perimenopause is usually indicated if you have the typical symptoms and you're over 45 years old, and there are no other underlying health considerations that could be causing the symptoms.

EARLY MENOPAUSE

For some women, menopause happens early, before the age of 45

Early menopause can happen naturally in some women, particularly if it runs in the family. This is sometimes called 'premature ovarian failure' and can be caused by an autoimmune disease, chromosome abnormalities or some infections – although in most cases there won't be an easily identifiable reason. However, not all early menopause is natural. Having a hysterectomy to remove your womb, for example, will lead to an immediate surgical menopause. Another reason why you might have an early menopause is if you have to undergo cancer treatment for some cancers.

Whatever the reason, early menopause can carry an increased risk of osteoporosis, meaning that hormone replacement therapies may be recommended if suitable. You may also be offered a bone protection medicine to help maintain bone density. If you're especially young, you may want to access counselling to help talk through the loss of fertility or other issues that might come up as a result of an early menopause.

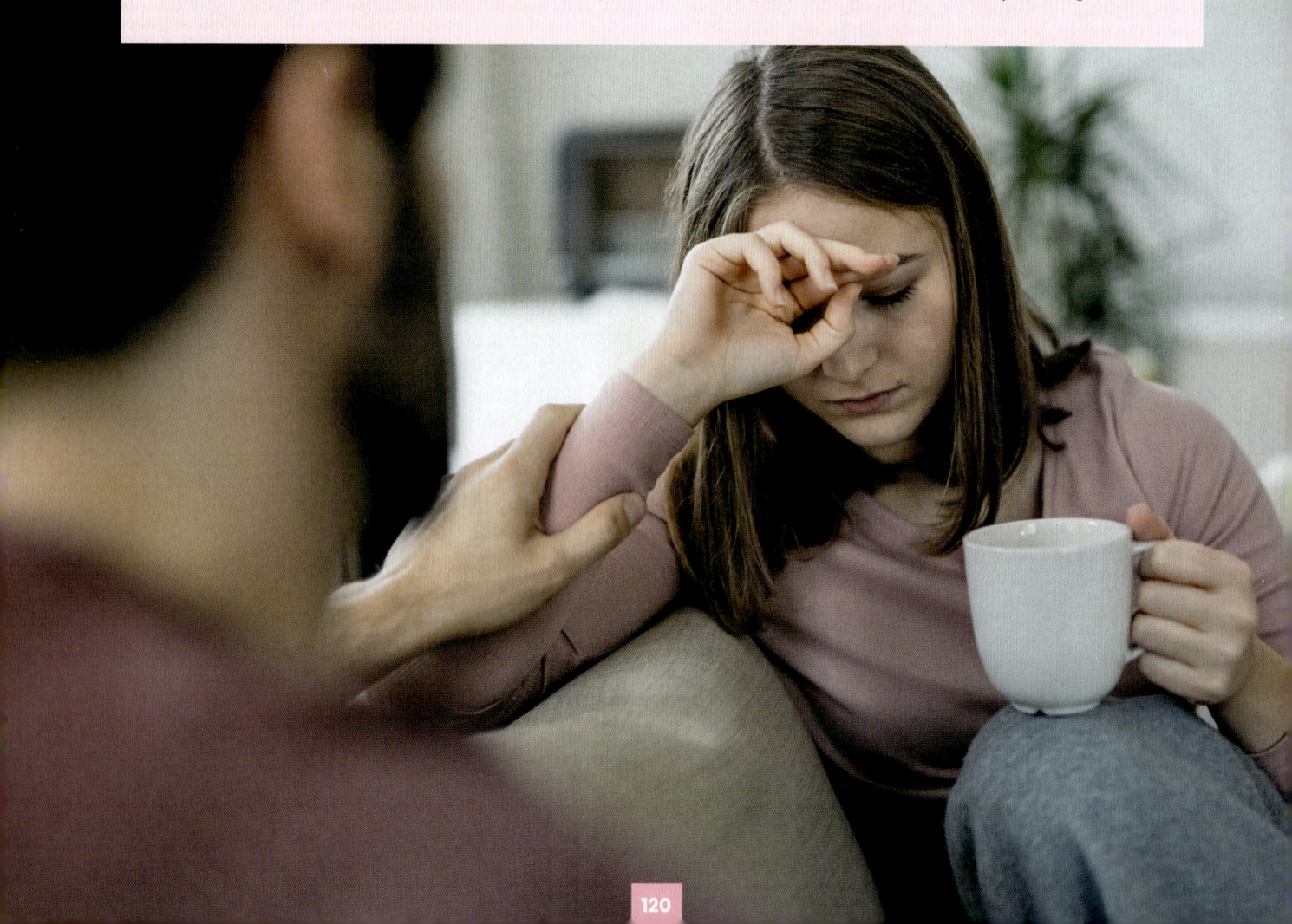

The final stage of menopause is everything that comes after your periods stop – post-menopause. This phase lasts for the rest of your life. There used to be a stereotype that a woman's life was more or less over when they reached menopause. But these days we live much longer, and post-menopause can last for 25 to 30 years and beyond. Not only that, many women find this stage is their best yet, as they have more independence and freedom than ever before. With a healthy lifestyle, you can feel fit, strong and well throughout this period.

COMMON SYMPTOMS

The main symptom of menopause is a change to your periods. In the earlier stages of perimenopause, it's not unusual to have shorter cycles, and then in the later stages, much longer ones. You may also start to have cycles where you don't ovulate at all. Not everyone has irregular periods as a first symptom of perimenopause. If you're on hormonal contraception, for example, this controls your cycle and you have a withdraw bleed, rather than a true period – and so you won't know if your natural cycle is disrupted.

POST-MENOPAUSAL POPULATION
In 2021, women aged 50 and over accounted for 26% of all women and girls around the world.[2]

> **"SLEEP IS OFTEN DISRUPTED, WHICH MIGHT BE DUE TO THE HIGHER LEVELS OF ANXIETY"**

Hot flushes and night sweats – collectively called vasomotor symptoms – are incredibly common. This is caused by the blood vessels dilating, causing more blood to rush through. This heat spreads through the body regardless of the external temperature, and can cause your face to flush and your body to sweat. Hot flushes can happen at any time and seem to come out of the blue. Night sweats are hot flushes that happen at night. They may have no cause, but sometimes you can identify triggers that make hot flushes worse. This includes things like caffeine, smoking, alcohol, spicy foods and stress.

You might feel more emotional than usual and have erratic mood swings. This is due to changing hormones, in the same way that adolescents might struggle to control their emotions during puberty. You might find that you're more irritable, snappy and frustrated than usual, finding it harder to cope in difficult situations. Many women also report they are more anxious around this time, even if they've never suffered with anxiety before.

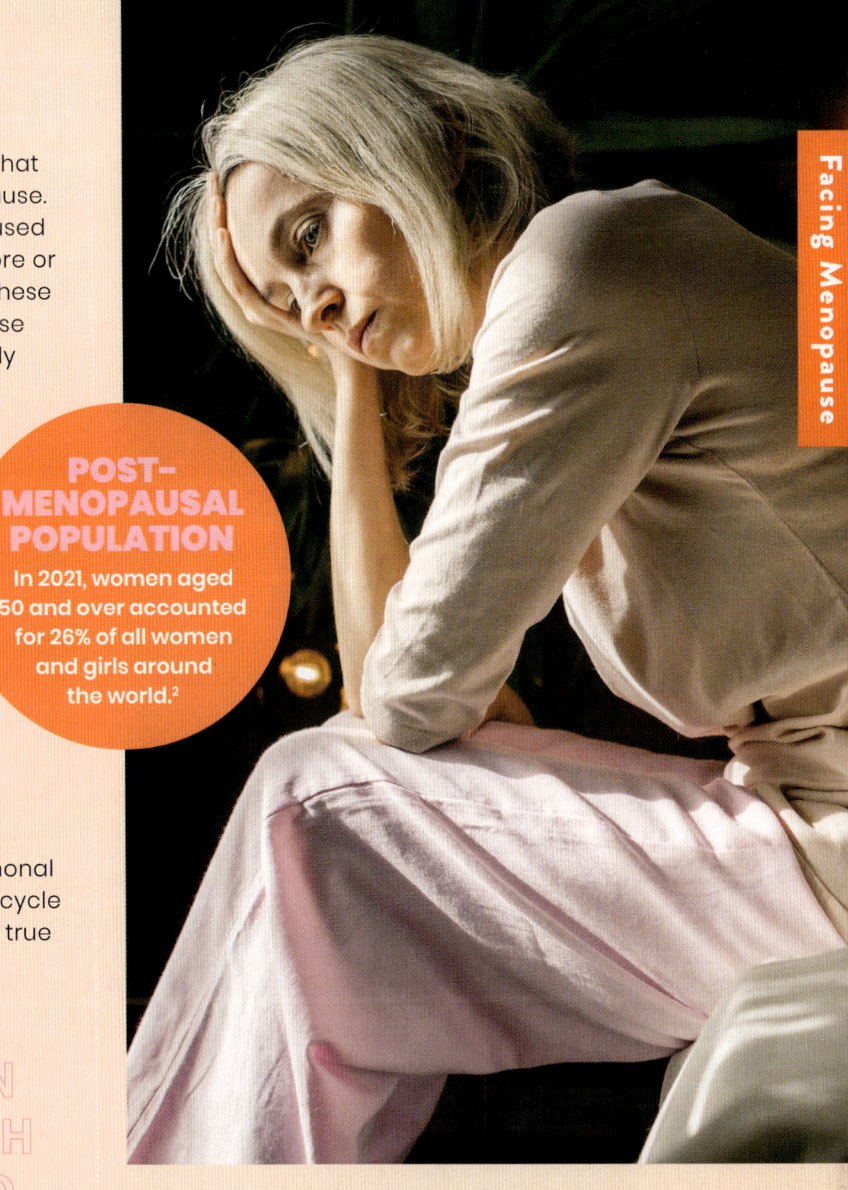

Oestrogen helps to retain bone and cartilage health, so as levels begin to drop, you might find that you get more headaches, joint pain and stiffness. You may also experience cramps and pains in your stomach, similar to period pains, as well as digestive issues. It's very common to experience vaginal dryness too, as oestrogen helps with lubrication, and this can lead to pain during sex. Sleep is often disrupted in perimenopause, which might be due to the higher levels of anxiety and stress, the night sweats or a new occurrence of insomnia. Your energy levels may be lower and you might feel more fatigued than usual. Many women report a lack of focus and concentration, as well as a general brain fog.

It can feel very hard when you're in the middle of it, but perimenopause doesn't last forever. Once you go through menopause and come out the other side, your hormone levels will stabilise at their new lower levels and your symptoms will taper off as your body adjusts.

HOW THE BODY CHANGES

As well as experiencing these physical and mental challenges, your body will begin to change. It's not unusual for women to gain a little weight at this time and for your body shape to also shift. You may start to hold on to more fat around the belly area, rather than it being more evenly distributed throughout the body.

Even if you change nothing about your current exercise routine and diet, you may see a small amount of weight gain. It's normal to gain weight as you age. This is due to multiple factors, such as a decline in muscle mass and a slowing metabolism. You might also find that you're simply busier with work and home life, especially if you're juggling children or older parents, and you don't have the time to exercise as much as you'd like or cook as often.

Oestrogen is an important factor in our metabolism, so the changes in our hormones can impact on appetite and the way we process and store fat. We also need oestrogen to maintain muscle mass; from the age of 40, we begin to lose muscle mass year on year. With less muscle, we don't need as much energy from our foods, which is another reason that we might see a little extra weight gain.

At the same time, our bone density starts to decline. This can make us more prone to bone breakages and fractures, and our risk of osteoporosis in later life becomes more significant.

In order to prevent this loss of bone density and muscle mass, we need to be proactive about our diet and exercise, making sure that we're eating plenty of calcium-rich foods and lean protein, and ensuring that we're doing enough weight-bearing strength exercise.

TREATMENT OPTIONS

There are two main approaches to managing the symptoms of menopause: medical or natural. The menopause transition isn't a hormone deficiency or a medical problem that we need to correct – it's completely natural and normal to go through. However, treatment is designed to help manage the symptoms and make the transition more tolerable, but you're under no pressure to go one way or another.

> "MENOPAUSE ISN'T A HORMONE DEFICIENCY OR A MEDICAL PROBLEM"

Hormone replacement therapy (HRT) has been around for a while now and can be very effective. It's a way of replacing the hormones lost through the natural process of menopause, boosting your levels and helping with any symptoms. It doesn't prevent menopause from happening, or prolong it; when you stop taking it, your hormone levels will be what they would have been if you hadn't taken it at all. For women who have a surgical menopause at a younger age, HRT is usually offered to help boost hormone levels and reduce the risk of certain health conditions that are more common after menopause. HRT is generally considered to be quite safe, but there are women for whom it might not be suitable. For example, if you have a history of certain cancers, such as breast, ovarian or womb, you may be advised not to take HRT at all, particularly if these were hormone-based cancers. You may also not be able to take HRT if you have a history of blood clots, untreated high blood pressure or liver disease.

Usually, you will begin with a low dose, and this is gradually increased to find the right level for you. It can be taken as a tablet, but more commonly is applied to the skin via a gel, spray or patch. There are different types of HRT, most commonly a combined oestrogen and progestogen. If you have a womb, taking oestrogen on its own can cause the lining of the uterus to thicken and increase the chance of endometrial or womb cancer. For those who don't have a womb (after a hysterectomy, for

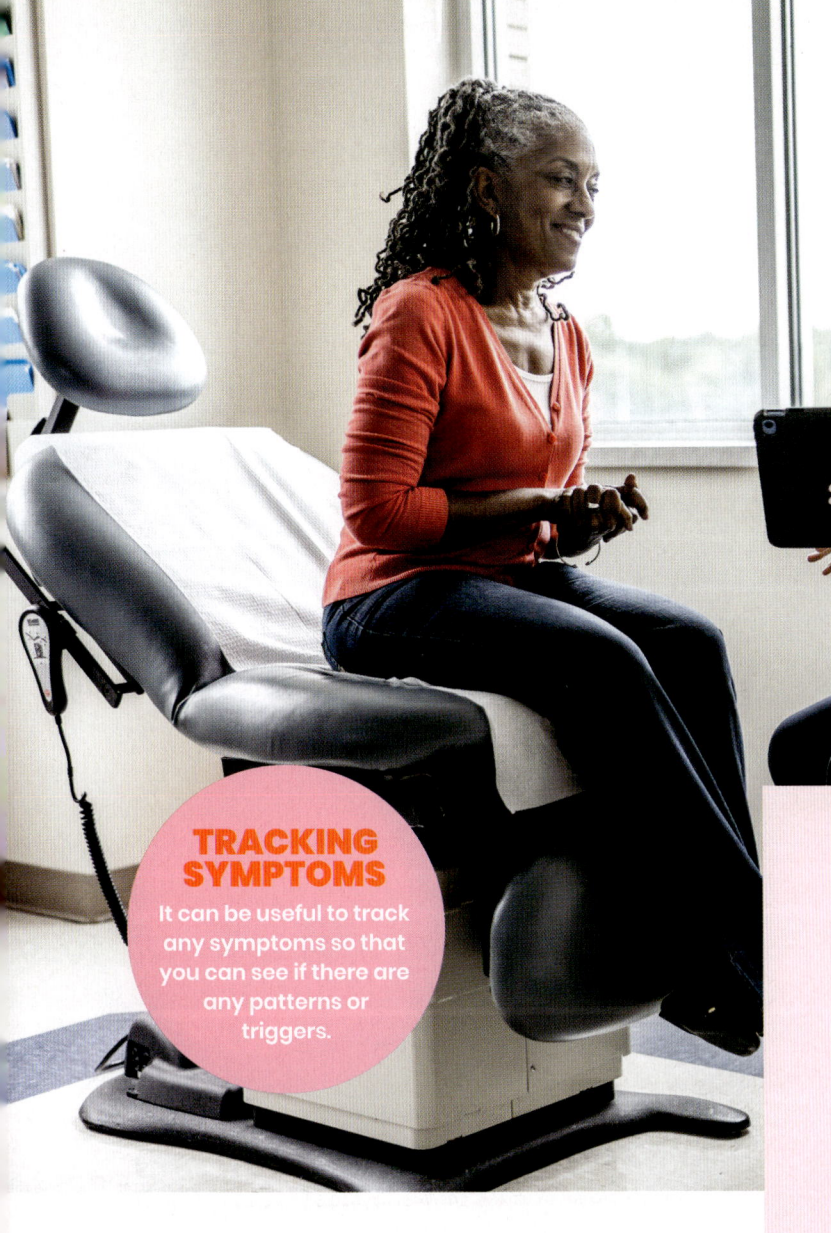

TRACKING SYMPTOMS
It can be useful to track any symptoms so that you can see if there are any patterns or triggers.

LESS COMMON SYMPTOMS

Perimenopause can affect you in lots of different ways that you might not expect

example), then oestrogen-only may be suitable. The exception is vaginal oestrogen, which is prescribed to only treat vaginal symptoms. It doesn't impact the whole body, which means that it is not necessary to take progestogen as well.

HRT is not the only option, and many women might choose not to or cannot have HRT. There are other medical options that treat individual symptoms. These include vasodilators, which help with vasomotor symptoms, certain anti-depressants that can be used off-label to help with hot flushes, and creams to ease vaginal dryness.

Lifestyle changes can also have a big impact on your symptoms, as well as reducing your risk of heart disease and some cancers, protecting your bones, reducing stress, and improving your mental health. This can also be partnered with a healthy, balanced diet, adding in more fruits and vegetables and reducing your intake of ultra-processed foods. It's a good idea to reduce your alcohol intake and stop smoking – both of these can increase your risk of certain cancers, impact on your risk of osteoporosis, and worsen perimenopausal symptoms. If you are overweight, bringing that down into a healthier weight range can also help with symptom control.

There are thought to be more than 30 recognised symptoms of perimenopause, some more common than others. You won't experience them all, but you might have a combination of many different ones. Some people find that they get tinnitus, for example, which can be particularly bad at night. You might get more dryness on your skin and in your mouth – even around your eyes! Your teeth and jaw can be affected by the drop in bone density, and your gumline could start to recede. Your hormones can play havoc with your gut microbiome and leave it feeling unbalanced. This can lead to digestive issues such as constipation, bloating or sensitivities to certain foods. Oestrogen can help to protect your urinary tract too, which means that you may have more UTIs or experience stress incontinence. All these symptoms can be treated in different ways – you don't have to suffer in silence.

HEART HEALTH
POST-MENOPAUSE

Look after your heart to enjoy a healthy, long and enjoyable later life

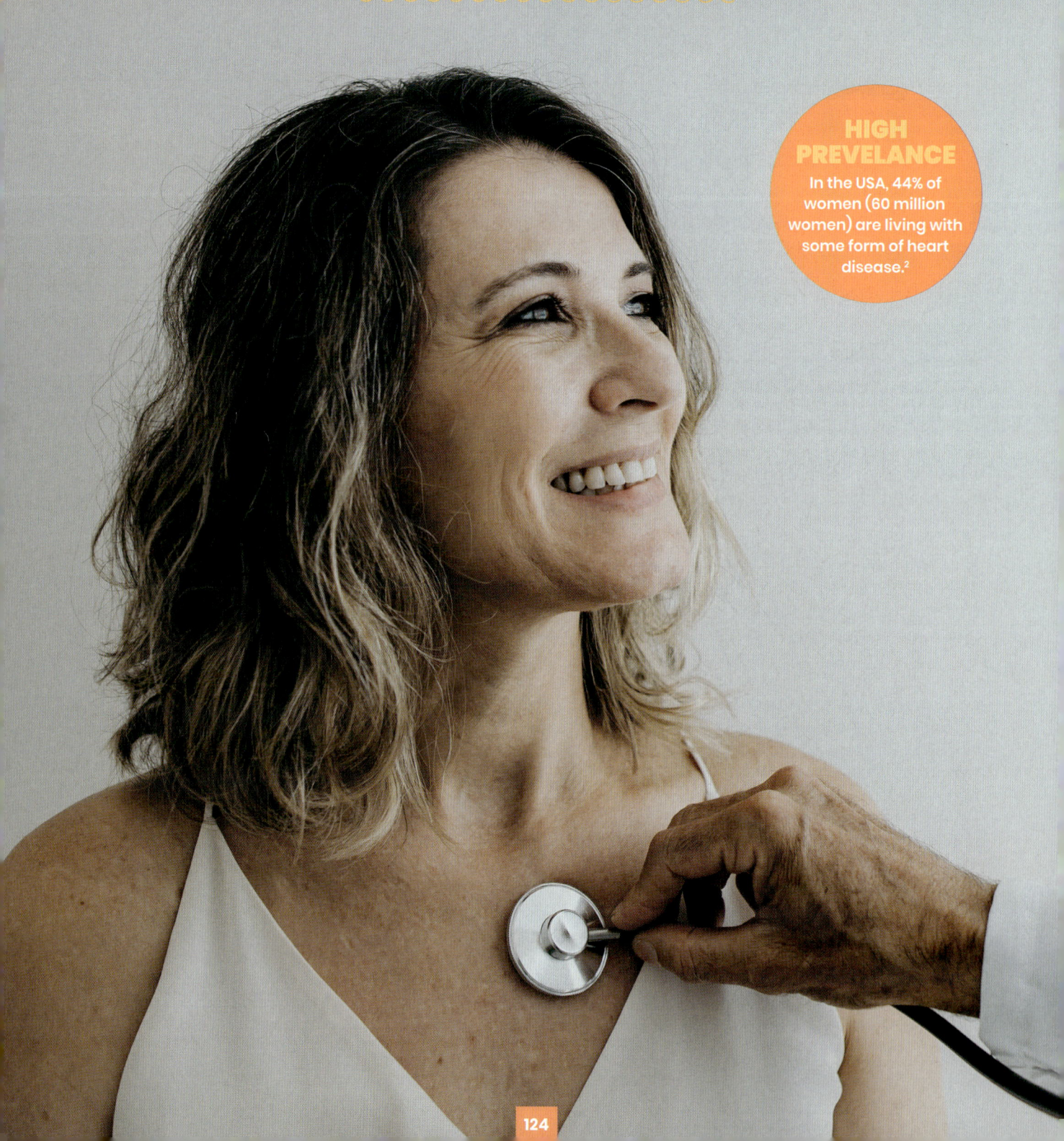

HIGH PREVELANCE

In the USA, 44% of women (60 million women) are living with some form of heart disease.[2]

Your cardiovascular health is important throughout your life, but even more so as you enter your post-menopause era. This is because your risk of heart disease increases once you have finished your reproductive years, due to losing the protective effect of oestrogen. Up until menopause, women are less likely to have a heart attack than a man of the same age, but after menopause, that is no longer the case. Cardiovascular disease is the leading cause of premature death for women globally.

When our oestrogen levels drop, lots of other changes can happen in our body that are also risk factors for heart disease. This includes high blood pressure, high cholesterol levels and high blood sugar levels. Our body composition can also change as our lean muscle mass begins to decrease. We might also put on a little weight, and we know that being overweight is a risk factor for heart disease. Lower energy levels might mean we're not exercising as much as we did before, which again is another risk factor, as is not getting enough sleep. If you experience vasomotor symptoms during menopause, such as hot flushes and night sweats, this can be a risk factor for heart disease too.[1]

HOW TO PROTECT YOUR HEART

If you're able to take it, then using HRT during perimenopause can help with many of the symptoms that can cause a rise in risk factors. It may offer protection against cardiovascular disease as a side effect, though HRT itself is not always suitable for women who already have cardiovascular symptoms or have a high risk of heart disease.

> "CARDIOVASCULAR DISEASE IS MOSTLY PREVENTABLE WITH THE RIGHT CHOICES"

It's more important to ensure that you're looking after yourself and adapting your lifestyle to protect your heart post-menopause. If you already live a heart-healthy lifestyle, then you will have gone a long way towards heart protection in your later life, but if you haven't, then it's never too late to make changes.

Maintaining a healthy weight is one of the best things you can do to keep your heart healthy. If you're overweight, then it can be hard to try to lose weight. You don't want to suddenly try a super-restrictive diet or intense exercise regime, which can both put extra strain on your heart. Rather, it's better to make small and sustainable changes. This should be a combination of a healthy, balanced diet and regular, physical exercise. Make sure that you're eating lots of heart-healthy foods, such as fruits and vegetables, wholegrains, healthy fats and lean protein, while limiting the foods that are high in fat and sugar. It doesn't really matter what exercise you do, as long as you enjoy it so that you keep doing it regularly. Not smoking, drinking plenty of water, limiting alcohol, and working to reduce stress can also help to lower your risk.

Cardiovascular disease is mostly preventable if you make the right lifestyle choices. The sooner you start to incorporate these into your day-to-day schedule, the quicker you can lower your risk of serious complications and the longer you can enjoy your post-menopause life. ■

MONITOR YOUR HEART HEALTH

Important check-ups you must have to look after your heart

BLOOD PRESSURE
You should keep an eye on your blood pressure, as hypertension is one of the main risk factors for heart disease. Most people don't know if their blood pressure is high unless they have it checked. You could get a machine for at home to keep an eye on your numbers, or have it checked with your doctor regularly.

CHOLESTEROL TESTS
You won't know if you have high cholesterol without having it checked. It's a simple finger-prick test and you get the results there and then. You can do this at your doctor's surgery or a pharmacy. It's advised to get a cholesterol test every four to six years.

HEIGHT, WEIGHT AND WAIST MEASUREMENT
These metrics help to determine your Body Mass Index (BMI), which isn't the perfect system as it doesn't take into account muscle mass, but it can give you an indication of whether you're a healthy weight. Your waist measurement is another guide – a waist-to-height ratio of above 0.5 indicates a higher risk of heart disease.

BONE & JOINT HEALTH

It's important to take steps to protect your bones and joints, especially when you're reaching menopause age

Oestrogen plays a vital role in the growth of healthy bones and preventing bone loss. It also has an anti-inflammatory effect, which can protect our joints. As we head into perimenopause and menopause, our oestrogen levels lower, which means that we lose these protective benefits.

PROBLEMS WITH BONE AND JOINT HEALTH

As we get older, our bone density starts to decline, bone formation is reduced and we have a higher risk of fractures, particularly in the hips and knees. We might also start to get more pain in our joints due to changes in the joint tissue. Muscle mass declines as we age as well, which means that the supporting muscles for the joints are less effective. If you also put on weight during menopause, this can place additional strain on the bones and joints.

All together, this leaves us with a higher risk of developing bone and joint conditions. Osteoporosis is a condition that weakens the bones, making them more likely to break. It develops slowly and we might only realise that we have the condition after breaking a bone. Osteoarthritis is a joint condition that makes the joints become painful and inflamed. It's more common in women than men, and more likely as we get older.

LOOKING AFTER YOUR BONES AND JOINTS

It's best to take a proactive approach to looking after your bones and joints. If you are not yet at perimenopause age, then the sooner you start to incorporate lifestyle tweaks to support your body, the less the impact will be later on. However, if you're already at that age, you can still do a great deal to improve and maintain your bone and joint health.

If it's right for you, then taking HRT can have a protective effect by replacing the lost oestrogen. If you're at risk of lower bone density, especially if you've had an early menopause, already have bone loss, or you have a family history of bone problems, then you may be able to take a medicine called bisphosphonates, which help to improve bone density and to prevent further bone loss. Anti-inflammatory medicines can also help you with any joint pain.

What you do in your lifestyle can help a lot. If you exercise regularly, incorporating weight-bearing activity, this can keep your muscles strong and joints flexible, and maintain your bone health. Walking is a great, low-impact exercise that anyone can do, even if you already have bone or joint issues.

Alongside that, make sure that you are eating a healthy diet. This should include good sources of calcium, which is key for bone health. Calcium is present in dairy products, but it's also in leafy greens and fortified cereals and breads. You need vitamin D alongside this to help absorb the calcium, so if you're not getting enough sunlight, you may need to use a supplement.

The main takeaway is to start looking after your bones and joints straight away; the sooner you start, the greater the impact and the longer you will go without any problems.

> "WALKING IS A GREAT EXERCISE THAT ANYONE CAN DO, EVEN IF YOU ALREADY HAVE BONE OR JOINT ISSUES"

COMMON BREAKAGES
About one in two women over 50 will break a bone due to osteoporosis in the USA.[1]

DEXA SCAN

We explain what happens with this bone density test

A DEXA scan looks at your bone density using low-dose x-rays. This can assess your risk of developing osteoporosis or diagnose the condition. It can be useful for those who are under 50 with high risk factors, such as previous broken bones, smoking or early menopause; and for those over 50 who may be at risk of developing the disease. The scan is quick and easy to perform. You can stay clothed, though you will need to remove anything that has metal on. The scan table will be opened, and you'll lie on your back, keeping very still. The scanning arm will pass over your body; it comes quite close, but it won't touch you. It normally takes about 10 to 20 minutes. Your results are compared to the expected bone density for a healthy adult of your age, which can determine your risk level.

ALZHEIMER'S IN WOMEN

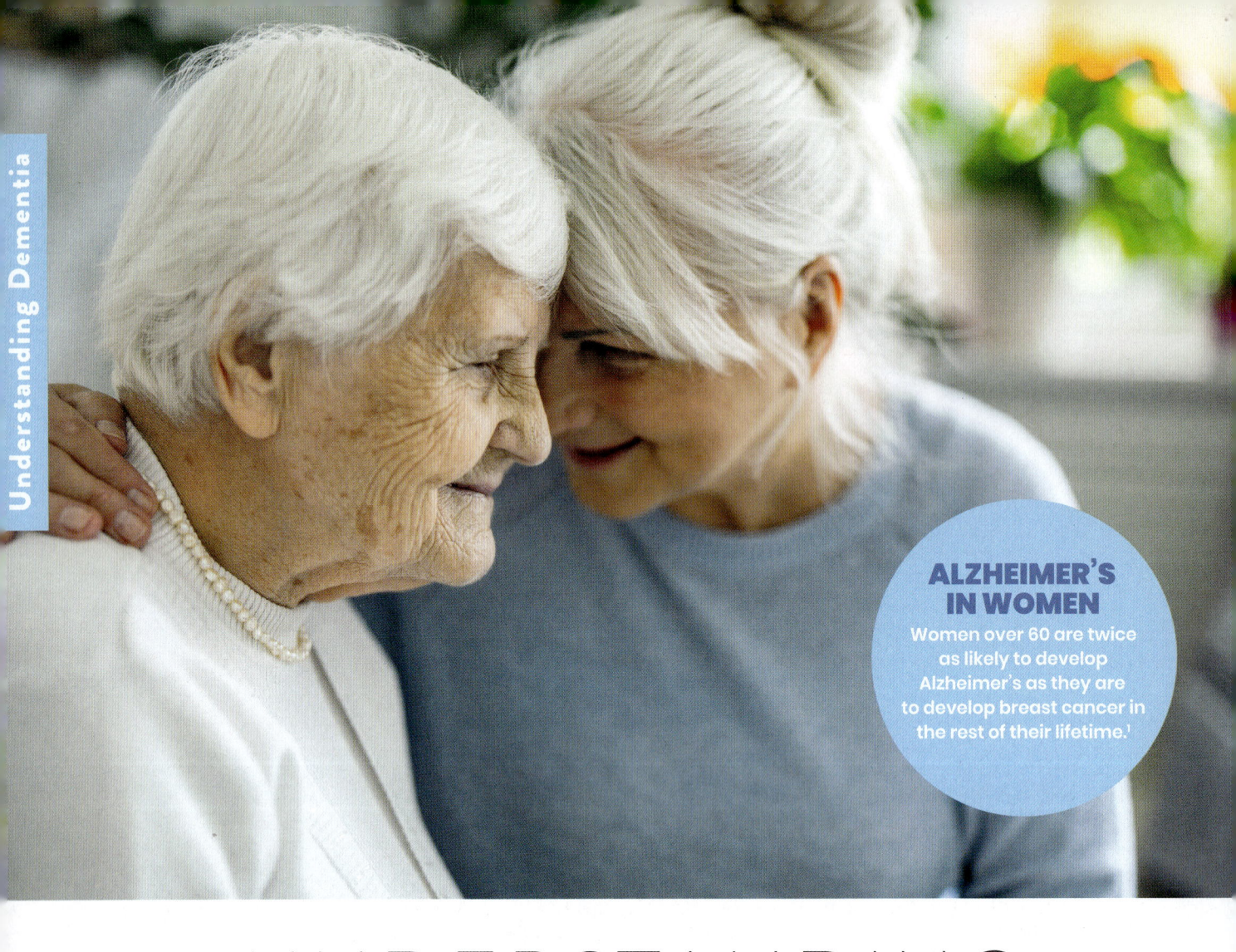

Women over 60 are twice as likely to develop Alzheimer's as they are to develop breast cancer in the rest of their lifetime.[1]

UNDERSTANDING DEMENTIA

Many of us are concerned about developing dementia in later life, but what is it and how can we reduce our risk?

Mental decline in later life is just as significant as physical decline. Anyone who has cared for someone with dementia will know how devastating this disease can be on both the person affected and those who love them.

Dementia is an umbrella term that encompasses several different symptoms that affect memory, cognitive ability, executive function, behaviour and language. As we get older, it's normal to start to be a little more forgetful than usual or to find it harder to concentrate. However, dementia is not a natural part of ageing, and the symptoms are life-changing and progressive. Dementia is a disease of the nerve cells in the brain, causing a decline in brain function.

There are many different types of dementia: 19 in 20 people with dementia will have one of the four

> **"EARLY SYMPTOMS CAN BE QUITE MILD, SO IT'S IMPORTANT TO VISIT A DOCTOR"**

main types, though the two most common are Alzheimer's disease and vascular dementia.

ALZHEIMER'S DISEASE

This is the most common cause of dementia. It's thought that as many as two-thirds of people living with dementia have Alzheimer's disease. The disease begins before any symptoms show – sometimes as much as 10 to 20 years before – causing damage in the brain through the build-up of substances that form a kind of plaque. The disease can affect everyone differently. The main symptoms include memory issues, problems with cognitive thinking and reasoning, language problems, and changes in mood and behaviours. The early symptoms can be quite mild, which is why it's important to visit a doctor if you're experiencing memory issues – it may be that there is another underlying reason, but it's better to know for sure. It can help to be diagnosed earlier as it gives you time to put in place the right support, find out more about the disease and its progression, and prepare yourself for what's to come. The symptoms will sadly get worse over time, and eventually someone with Alzheimer's disease will need support to engage in daily activities.

Women are more likely than men to develop Alzheimer's disease. In part, this is because women live longer than men, and age is the biggest risk factor in developing dementia. There isn't enough research yet exploring why women are so much more affected, but it's thought that hormonal changes could play a part. Oestrogen helps to maintain brain health, so it's possible that going through menopause impacts a woman's risk.

VASCULAR DEMENTIA

Vascular dementia is caused by a reduced blood flow to the brain, and it is progressive. Caught early enough, it is possible to slow down the progression of the disease. Symptoms include slower thoughts, difficulty with planning, problems with concentration, changes to mood, and difficulty with balance. It's not uncommon to have both vascular dementia and Alzheimer's disease. Vascular dementia can be caused by a narrowing of the blood vessels in the brain (which can be linked to some lifestyle risk factors), a stroke or a series of mini strokes (TIAs).

Once diagnosed, it's sadly not possible to reverse the damage done to the brain, but it is possible, with some lifestyle changes, to at least slow it down. This means eating a healthy diet, losing weight, not smoking or drinking too much, treating other health conditions like hypertension and high cholesterol, and doing problem-solving activities to keep the brain active.

REDUCING YOUR RISK

Lifestyle interventions can help reduce your risk of developing dementia in later life

Being in good health when you're younger can impact your risk of developing dementia. According to Alzheimer's Society, evidence shows that dementia risk is lower in those who have healthy behaviours during mid-life (40-65 years old). Here are the lifestyle factors that have the best chance of reducing your risk, though no one behaviour is better than others:

EXERCISE
Being physically active throughout your life can reduce your risk of developing dementia – ideally a combination of cardio work and strength training. If you're currently inactive, even starting to move a little more can have an impact.

MENTAL HEALTH
Those who have depression can be more at risk of developing dementia in later life, so ensure you're taking time to look after your mental wellbeing and seeking help if you do have mental health issues.

DIET
A healthy diet can help to lower your chance of long-term health problems like diabetes, high blood pressure and high cholesterol, which can all increase the risk of dementia.

ALCOHOL
If you regularly drink more than the recommended healthy limits, this can increase your risk of developing dementia.

THE HEALTHY WOMAN'S HANDBOOK

Future PLC Quay House, The Ambury, Bath, BA1 1UA

Editorial
Author **Julie Bassett**
Group Editor **Sarah Bankes**
Art Editor **Madelene King**
Head of Art & Design **Greg Whitaker**
Editorial Director **Jon White**
Managing Director **Grainne McKenna**

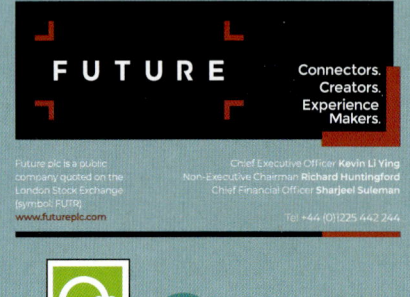

Contributor
Jayne Nelson

Cover images
© Getty Images

Photography
All copyrights and trademarks are recognised and respected

Advertising
Media packs are available on request
Commercial Director **Clare Dove**

International
Head of Print Licensing **Rachel Shaw**
licensing@futurenet.com

Circulation
Head of Newstrade **Tim Mathers**

Production
Head of Production **Mark Constance**
Production Project Manager **Matthew Eglinton**
Advertising Production Manager **Joanne Crosby**
Digital Editions Controller **Jason Hudson**
Production Managers **Keely Miller, Nola Cokely, Vivienne Calvert, Fran Twentyman**

Printed in the UK

Distributed by www.marketforce.co.uk
For enquiries, please email: mfcommunications@futurenet.com

GPSR EU RP (for authorities only)
eucomply OÜ Pärnu mnt 139b-14 11317, Tallinn, Estonia
hello@eucompliancepartner.com, +3375690241

The Healthy Woman's Handbook First Edition (LBZ7029)
© 2025 Future Publishing Limited

We are committed to only using magazine paper which is derived from responsibly managed, certified forestry and chlorine-free manufacture. The paper in this bookazine was sourced and produced from sustainable managed forests, conforming to strict environmental and socioeconomic standards.

All contents © 2025 Future Publishing Limited or published under licence. All rights reserved. No part of this magazine may be used, stored, transmitted or reproduced in any way without the prior written permission of the publisher. Future Publishing Limited (company number 2008885) is registered in England and Wales. Registered office: Quay House, The Ambury, Bath BA1 1UA. All information contained in this publication is for information only and is, as far as we are aware, correct at the time of going to press. Future cannot accept any responsibility for errors or inaccuracies in such information. You are advised to contact manufacturers and retailers directly with regard to the price of products/services referred to in this publication. Apps and websites mentioned in this publication are not under our control. We are not responsible for their contents or any other changes or updates to them. This magazine is fully independent and not affiliated in any way with the companies mentioned herein.

FUTURE Connectors. Creators. Experience Makers.

Future plc is a public company quoted on the London Stock Exchange (symbol: FUTR)
www.futureplc.com

Chief Executive Officer **Kevin Li Ying**
Non-Executive Chairman **Richard Huntingford**
Chief Financial Officer **Sharjeel Suleman**

Tel +44 (0)1225 442 244